Traumatic Brain Injury Rehabilitation

Practical Vocational, Neuropsychological, and Psychotherapy Interventions

edited by
Robert T. Fraser, Ph.D., C.R.C.
David C. Clemmons, Ph.D., C.R.C.

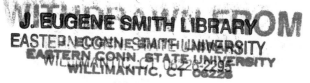

CRC Press
Boca Raton London New York Washington, D.C.

Library of Congress Cataloging-in-Publication Data

Traumatic brain injury rehabilitation : practical vocational, neuropsychological, and psychotherapy interventions / edited by Robert T. Fraser, David C. Clemmons.
    p. cm.
Includes bibliographical references and index.
ISBN 0-8493-3315-6
1. Brain damage--Patients--Rehabilitation. 2. Vocational
I. Fraser, Robert T. II. Clemmons, David Charles.
      [DNLM: 1. Brain injuries--rehabilitation. 2. Brain injuries-
-psychology. 3. Rehabilitation, Vocational--methods
4. Counseling. 5. Psychotherapy. WL 354 T77785 1999]
    RC387.5.T736 1999
    617.4'81044--dc21
                                    99-30237
                                        CIP

© 2000 by CRC Press LLC

No claim to original U.S. Government works
International Standard Book Number 0-8493-3315-6
Library of Congress Card Number 99-30237
Printed in the United States of America   2 3 4 5 6 7 8 9 0
Printed on acid-free paper

Foreword

The authors are well aware that there are many existing, fine texts related to traumatic brain injury rehabilitation. The emphasis or niche of this text, however, is a move toward the more practical or "how to" level of rehabilitation intervention which is often the challenge for members of the rehabilitation team or the sole field rehabilitation practitioner.

The editors are delighted to have had the contributions of key professionals in their area of expertise: Jay Uomoto, Keith Cicerone, C. Gerald Warren, Paul Wehman, Brian McMahon, and Rita Curl in the development of this work. These professionals, all of whom have academic affiliations, are unique in as much as they are individuals who have moved beyond a conceptual status to pilot and then refine effective psychosocial and vocational rehabilitation interventions for survivors of TBI within the community. The information provided within this text is gleaned not only from years of their combined experience, but from perspectives gathered from their exposure to centers throughout the country — we thank all who have contributed to our pool of experience and knowledge.

This book should be helpful not only to the neophyte rehabilitation practitioner in TBI rehabilitation, but also to the seasoned rehabilitation practitioner looking for new interventions or rehabilitation program ideas that can improve an organization's functional outcome. The range of topics covered (e.g., a functional emphasis in neuropsychological report writing, a framework for individual and group psychotherapy, a review of primarily low-cost assistive technology interventions, TBI vocational evaluation and placement systems, etc.) have direct application in daily service delivery for members of this rehabilitation population. The informational focus within this text is on its direct *relevancy* to the practitioner.

Where necessary, we have replaced the plural pronoun *their* with the singular, masculine pronoun "him" and its derivative "his" in order to facilitate grammatically correct sentences, allowing the pronoun to agree in number with the noun it replaces. The words "him" and "his" are, therefore, not used here to denote gender.

In addition to the collaborating authors, the editors would like to thank our friend Dennis McClellan of CRC Press who brought this project to us; Ms. Barbara Norwitz also of CRC Press whose "menacing eyes" and support promoted its completion; Mr. Tomm Munro, who diligently prepared and organized the book for submission to CRC; and to Hugh Fraser for his extra inspiration in "getting things done."

It should be noted that this text is an outgrowth of earlier training efforts supported by the U.S. Office of Special Education and Rehabilitation Services (OSERS, Grant No. H1129T80031-89) and current partial support of the University of Washington Traumatic Brain Injury Model Systems grant (H133A9800) awarded by the National Institute on Disability and Rehabilitation Research (NIDRR). All profits from the sale of this book are utilized within the University of Washington Department of Neurology for support of client vocational placement services (not grant-supported) or to provide rehabilitation training activities specific to traumatic brain injury rehabilitation.

Robert T. Fraser
David C. Clemmons
February, 1999

About the Editors

Robert T. Fraser, Ph.D., C.R.C. is a professor in the University of Washington's Department of Neurology, jointly with Neurosurgery and Rehabilitation Medicine. He is a counseling and rehabilitation psychologist and a certified rehabilitation counselor.

Dr. Fraser is author or co-author of more than sixty-five publications, in addition to a video series on traumatic brain injury rehabilitation. He has been awarded numerous federal grants by the Department of Education (NIDRR and RSA) — four of which have been specific to traumatic brain injury rehabilitation. He was awarded a World Rehabilitation Fund fellowship to review the post-acute traumatic brain injury programs in Israel and has received two American Rehabilitation Counseling Association Research Awards.

Dr. Fraser is a past president of Rehabilitation Psychology, Division 22 of the American Psychological Association and a Fellow in the Division (EFA), a former Board Member of the Epilepsy Foundation of America and recently appointed to the EFA Professional Advisory Board.

David C. Clemmons, Ph.D., C.R.C. is a counseling and rehabilitation psychologist and certified rahabilitation counselor. He earned a doctorate in rehabilitation psychology from the University of Washington in 1985 and received Washington state psychology licensure in 1987.

His professional interests include the development of vocational rehabilitation and counseling strategies for persons with central nervous system disease. He has been investigator or co-investigator on seven major federally funded rehabilitation grants and demonstration projects in the past twelve years.

Dr. Clemmons has authored and co-authored many publications in neurological rehabilitation, including a new video/monograph series on counseling strategies for persons with impairment in brain function. He regularly presents one- to three-day training symposia nationally in the field of neurological vocational rehabilitation.

Dr. Clemmons is presently Director of Vocational Services at the University of Washington Regional Epilepsy Center.

Contributors

John Bricout, Ph.D.
Assistant Professor
School of Social Work
Washington University
St. Louis, Washington

Keith D. Cicerone, Ph.D.
Director of Neuropsychology
Center for Head Injuries
JFK - Hardwick at Oaktree
Edison, New Jersey
Associate Professor of Neurosciences
Seton Hall University
West Orange, New Jersey

Rita Curl, Ph.D.
Professor, Department of Psychology
Director of Research
North Dakota Center for Disabilities
Minot State University
Minot, North Dakota

Brian T. McMahon, Ph.D., C.R.C.
Professor and Chair
Department of Rehabilitation Counseling
Virgina Commonwealth University
Richmond, Virginia

Pam Targett, M.Ed.
Director of Employment Services
Rehabilitation Research and Training Center
Virginia Commonwealth University
Richmond, Virginia

Jay M. Uomoto, Ph.D.
Associate Professor and Director of Research
Department of Psychology
Seattle Pacific University
Seattle, Washington

C. Gerald Warren, MPA
President, C. Gerald Warren and Associates
Clinical Professor
University of Washington
Department of Rehabilitation Medicine and Center for Bioengineering
Seattle, Washington

Paul Wehman, Ph.D.
Professor of Rehabilitation
Medicine and Special Education
Medical College of Virginia
Richmond, Virginia

Dedication

This book is dedicated to the courageous efforts of survivors of traumatic brain injury as they strive to achieve productive lives, and to the committed rehabilitation professionals who assist them in this challenge.

Contents

chapter one

Application of the neuropsychological evaluation in vocational planning after brain injury

Jay M. Uomoto, Ph.D.

Introduction

Traumatic brain injury (TBI) continues to result in disability that requires comprehensive and often lengthy rehabilitation efforts. It is costly from the standpoint of rehabilitation costs, lost earnings, and therefore, loss to the gross national product, but moreover, costly from the human suffering viewpoint. Health-care professionals are continually challenged in their efforts to return those with TBI to the workforce. The major thrust of this chapter is to educate rehabilitation professionals on the role of the neuropsychological evaluation as a tool in assisting those with TBI to return to work. The chapter is intended for the broad audience of professionals who work with individuals with TBI who may appropriately utilize the data generated through a neuropsychological evaluation.

From the moment of injury to the first day of employment after TBI, there is often a long and arduous process of treatment and therapies that prepare a person for returning to activities that approximate pre-injury experiences. There is no typical length of TBI rehabilitation. Much depends on the severity level of the TBI, the nature and extent of problems, availability of social support networks, accessible and available appropriate rehabilitation, and the circumstances surrounding re-employment and the community job market. Outcomes of rehabilitation efforts span a wide range. Fewer individuals return to work at the same level, for the same pay, and at the same number of hours per week as before the injury. Some return to a similar job at a full- to part-time level, with a reduced rate of pay. Many are totally and permanently disabled from ever working again in a competitive setting. These individuals may seek volunteer positions or pursue a vocational interests. Psychosocial outcomes encompass a similar range, from those being able to resume a familiar social and family life to those who become divorced or separated, or experience shrinking social networks.

In the context of this chapter, the task before rehabilitation professionals is to maximize the potential of the individual with brain injury to return to as high a level of pre-injury productivity as can be achieved. Further efforts in rehabilitation may focus upon establishing new and different life goals and activities. The goal of rehabilitation, therefore, involves an enormous effort on the part of both the patient and rehabilitation personnel. Hopefully, the following will provide a good working knowledge of neuropsychological assessment so that the reader will be able to utilize test findings to better the employment outcome for this population.

It is well beyond the scope of this chapter to thoroughly review the field of clinical neuropsychology. It is an ever-expanding discipline with research findings that are constantly changing the field. Interested readers are encouraged to investigate other texts, journal articles, and resources that can provide greater depth and breadth for the field as a whole. Appendix A is an annotated bibliography of some neuropsychological resources that may provide further references for more in-depth study.

Neuropsychology as the study of brain-behavior relationships

One of the earliest uses of the term *neuropsychology* was recorded in a lecture delivered at the Phipps Psychiatric Clinic at Johns Hopkins University in 1913 by the famous humanitarian physician, Sir William Osler.[1] It was Dr. Osler's hope that a new field be developed whose focus was to train students in neuropsychology as a means to better understand the issues of mental illness.

In a standard text by Kolb and Whishaw,[2] the authors note that neuropsychology as a unified field of study has only been recognized as a distinctive area of the general field of psychology since the mid-1970s. As with many fields of study within psychology, neuropsychology has basic science, animal, and human experimental research realms, as well as a clinical application arm. There are other fields that overlap neuropsychology that are worth mentioning to provide some clarity. The emerging field of cognitive neuroscience (see Rugg[3] for an overview) is a related field that deals with formulating biopsychosocial models of cognition. It is an interdisciplinary field that includes cognitive psychology, neurology, neuroscience, experimental psychology, computer science, and several other disciplines that focus on understanding human cognitive functioning. Behavioral neurology[4,5] is another field closely related to neuropsychology in that its main focus is on brain function and dysfunction relative to impairments in thinking and behavior. Neuropsychiatry can be seen to overlap neuropsychology since it is concerned with psychiatric disorders that have bases in neurological substrates.

The focus of the present discussion will be those aspects of neuropsychology that deal with assessment and treatment based upon brain–behavior relationships. The term *clinical* in clinical neuropsychology underscores the reality that human function exists within a biopsychosocial context (see Engel[6] and Paris[7] for an explication of the biopsychosocial model). That is, one cannot understand human behavior unless its related biological underpinnings, psychological processes, and social or interpersonal levels of analysis are considered.

Neuropsychology is a systematic way of examining the relationship between what occurs at the biological level in the brain and what a person does behaviorally. Human behavior is extremely complex; even seemingly simple actions, such as looking at a telephone number in the yellow pages to dial for a pizza delivery, may be complex. You first scan the telephone number from left to right. This is based upon an overlearned skill (called procedural memory) that allows you to apply the "left to right" rule to this particular situation. Attention to this number takes place and numbers must be recognized as being numbers (versus letters or just random blots of ink). The set of numbers that are read must then be stored in both verbal and visual memory, while at the same time keeping in mind the type of pizza you wish to order. You then begin briefly rehearsing the sequence of numbers to be punched on a touch-tone telephone. Since a telephone call is being placed, some decision may be required to determine whether or not to use a certain prefix area code. Once the prefix is determined, you may need to decide if it's a long distance number, in which case a "1" must be entered prior to the area code. You continue to rehearse the original seven to ten digits as you begin punching in the numbers on the keypad of your telephone, while continuing to keep in visual memory the type of pizza you wished to order.

Note, too, that the pizza order itself is multidimensional and includes the size of pizza, type of crust, and the listing of toppings. Unless you are talking on the telephone in a completely silent room without any visual distractions, there will be the additional cognitive demand of focusing one's attention on the voice of the person on the other end of the telephone line. Your ability to filter out television stimuli or ambient room noise and focus on the rather faint voice of the person on the line (bearing in mind that you have the receiver only on one ear) may be influenced by the amount of sleep you had the night before, your degree of hunger at the moment, and other physical states. Psychological stressors, such as knowing you are trying to meet an important business deadline, may influence your ability to focus on this telephone call. Visual imagery likely engages as soon as you hear the person's voice. Here, you are pulling up from long-term storage images of people and contexts that may be consistent with the actual situation of the person at the pizza restaurant, while at the same time constructing intelligible verbiage to convey the purposes of your call.

All of these cognitive events occur within a span of a few seconds; some occur within microseconds. The task of neuropsychology is to analyze these various aspects and sequences of cognition relative to meaningful everyday functioning. The neuropsychological evaluation attempts to capture, in snapshot fashion, the cognitive functioning status of a particular individual. This individual is evaluated within the context of specific physical and biological states. These states may be influenced by a particular set of psychosocial stressors that modify the particular cognitive capacity of that individual.

Many behaviorally oriented psychologists will maintain that there is no such thing as undetermined behavior. From a neuropsychological point of view, this also holds true. Any action that is produced by human beings corresponds to some event that occurs in the brain. While a neurologist, a physiologist, or radiologist may spend their careers examining the intricate substrates of the brain matter itself, neuropsychologists spend most of their day making observations on human behavior and drawing conclusions about what caused those behaviors. What determines a particular behavior can be viewed on several levels. Figure 1 depicts the several realms of data that a neuropsychologist will examine to assist in making sense of particular behaviors.

If a client with TBI is observed being late to work, the neuropsychologist may be asked to judge to what degree memory impairment contributes to this person's problem with timeliness. In this case, the neuropsychologist would need to know the extent of brain injury (brain physiology) as determined by diagnostic imaging (CT or MRI scan) and/or electrodiagnostic measures (EEG). There may be physical barriers to timeliness (e.g., gait disorder, balance problems, weakness on one side of the body) which make commuting or getting ready for work in the morning a more time-consuming process. Fatigue and sleep problems after brain injury may slow a person's morning routine, thus making him late to work. Simple observations can be made regarding lack of promptness for a neuropsychological testing appointment or if when conversing with a client, you notice that your name is quickly forgotten (direct observations). Memory tests may be given to assess both verbal and visual retention skills. Tests of attention and concentration may also be given (specific neuropsychological testing).

Inquiries into any interpersonal conflicts on the job, perhaps with a supervisor or co-worker who the client expects to see in the morning, may assist in the evaluation (interpersonal actions). It can be determined if this is an individual who is simply "laid back" vs. depressed which may make the person lethargic and sluggish at the work site (based upon personality functioning test data). Gathering information regarding the client's litigation status may shed light on the picture. For example, does a client stand to lose compensation by "looking too functional" on the job? Are there others in a client's social network who may have a stake in how well a person functions at home, in the community, or in a work situation (attorney, spouse, or employer)?

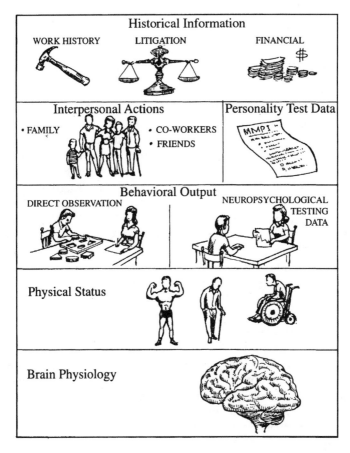

Figure 1   Realms of data that are pertinent in a neuropsychological evaluation.

Information about work history (historical information) can help complete the clinical picture. For example, did the person always arrive late prior to injury, or is this a new behavior? Rarely is there a single explanation for a given behavior and it is most often a combination of several of the above factors. Determining the factors that significantly contribute to a problem may assist the health care professional and, particularly the vocational counselor, in solving the problem at hand. In this case, the vocational counselor identifies the timeliness problem as being due primarily to poor organizational routines and short-term memory problems concerning the bus schedule. The counselor may then find a therapist to work with the client on use of a memory book and establish a morning organizational routine (e.g., an occupational therapist may be called for case consultation).

In sum, the study of the relationship between brain functioning and behavioral output is the primary content of neuropsychology. The neuropsychological evaluation is a method of examining this relationship. It should be noted here that there is a difference between a neuropsychological evaluation and neuropsychological testing. Testing is just one part of an evaluation.

Psychological and neuropsychological testing

Many neuropsychologists will also conduct a clinical interview with the client for diagnostic and background information. Often a collateral source, such as a family member, friend, employer, or co-worker is also interviewed. This is important since the person with brain injury may not be fully aware of the nature and range of cognitive or neurobehavioral problems that are exhibited in the home or community. Medical and other records are reviewed. A thorough examination of the medical findings and opinions can provide needed information to put into perspective how far the client has progressed from the time of injury. Emotional status and personality factors are also important variables to consider in neuropsychological assessment. To augment neuropsychological testing, an evaluation generally includes the administration of a standardized personality inventory, such as the Minnesota Multiphasic Personality Inventory (MMPI, MMPI-2) or the Millon Clinical Multiaxial Inventory (MCMI-I, II, III). The impact of personality and emotional variables on neurological status is discussed later in this chapter.

In neuropsychological testing, the neuropsychologist or a trained examiner (referred to as a psychometrist) administers and scores standardized tests of cognitive functioning. The use of standardized tests is essential for obtaining reliable and valid results. The tests that are utilized in a flexible or fixed battery method, therefore, should possess excellent psychometric characteristics of reliability and validity. The reliability of a test refers to the degree of consistency of test scores produced by an individual on repeat examinations. On a test with 100% reliability, a person would always earn exactly the same score on successive examinations, assuming, of course, that the person had not changed. This would be a rare event, but it is important that neuropsychological tests be as consistent as possible. High reliability ensures accurate documentation of recovery or loss of functioning on successive testings. Reliability also sets the upper limits on another important psychometric concept, that of validity.

Validity refers to the degree to which a test actually assesses the concept it is intended to measure. Neuropsychological tests used to measure similar traits (e.g., memory, problem-solving ability) must have good concurrent validity. Another important attribute for neuropsychological tests is that of predictive validity: the degree to which one may make predictions of future or concurrent behavior based on a test result. This is critical for neuropsychological evaluations because the utility of these evaluations is to make inferences regarding real-life behaviors such as competitive employability or success at a particular work task. A related concept is that a neuropsychological test must possess ecological validity. This is similar to predictive validity in that a test should be able to inform the neuropsychologist of what a client's behavior in the community will actually be, based upon the pattern of results. Often, single tests of a particular cognitive function will not necessarily have high ecological validity if interpreted in isolation. However, that same test result, if reviewed within the context of a set of measures and observations, will be more instructive relative to a person's daily functioning.

Neuropsychological testing samples a person's behavior in a structured setting. The testee sits in a quiet room in which the examiner sits opposite and administers a set of standardized neuropsychological tests. These tests are then scored and interpreted by a neuropsychologist. Obtaining information in this manner is similar to taking soil samples to test the toxicity of soil underneath the foundation of a gas station with questionable underground tank leakage. One does not test all the soil, but obtains a representative sample of soil. In evaluating a person's thinking abilities, one does not test every possible aspect of thinking, but rather tries to assess an adequate range of brain–behavior relationships to make reasonable inferences about a person's functional abilities.

Purposes of the neuropsychological evaluation

There are basically five major purposes for obtaining a neuropsychological evaluation. Evaluations are usually requested for very specific reasons, and that purpose varies depending upon the setting and situation. The major purpose for conducting an evaluation is largely dependent upon the referral question and the specific circumstances under which the client must function. The five major purposes are (1) diagnostic, (2) treatment planning and monitoring, (3) discharge planning, (4) community functioning, and (5) vocational planning. In each of these areas, the documentation of areas of relative strength, as well as of cognitive deficit, is an important part of the evaluation.

Diagnostic

The neuropsychological evaluation is one method for obtaining information on the integrity of brain function. The sensitivity of tests refers to the degree to which tests are sensitive enough to detect brain dysfunction. Singular tests such as the Trailmaking Test (Part B), the Category Test, and the Stroop Color-Word Test are three examples of tests that are highly sensitive to the presence of brain dysfunction. They may not, however, be specific to the nature or type of neurological condition involved. The specificity of a test refers to the degree to which a test is specific to particular brain disorders or conditions. Few singular neuropsychological tests are specific to particular kinds of disorders, hence, the need for a more comprehensive approach is usually taken for the task of understanding *patterns* of *cognitive problems*, which, in turn, may be more specific to certain brain conditions.

The neuropsychological evaluation can also provide information on the general level of impairment. The neuropsychologist will estimate an individual's pre-injury level of cognitive abilities based upon age, educational attainment, and occupation. Mathematical equations can be employed to estimate pre-injury or premorbid long-term intellectual functioning levels. This is one index of pre-injury functioning by which a particular client's performance is compared and judged. Some tests on the neuropsychological evaluation are more robust and less apt to decline in mild to moderate severity levels of brain injury (e.g., Information and Vocabulary subtests of the Wechsler Adult Intelligence Scale). The general level of impairment and decline post-injury can be made based upon this pre-injury estimate. For example, assume a person possesses a pre-injury estimated level of cognitive functioning in the Average range (equivalent to I.Q. scores between 90 and 109). Later, that person sustains a brain injury in an accident and obtains neuropsychological test scores in the Low Average range. One can then hypothesize that there is evidence for mild cognitive impairment as a result of brain injury. If someone else is estimated to have a pre-injury cognitive level in the Very Superior range (I.Q. equivalence of 130 or greater) and then, after sustaining a brain injury, tested in the Superior range (I.Q. equivalent of 120), a similar conclusion could be made. This represents mild cognitive impairment, even though the actual scores are in the Superior range. There-fore, determining cognitive or intellectual deficits depends largely on a per-son's pre-injury level of abilities. For a review of different strategies that are utilized to determine pre-morbid cognitive and intellectual functioning, see Kareken;[8] Franzen, Burgess, and Smith-Seemiller;[9] Williams;[10] Hartlage;[11] and Reynolds.[12]

The neuropsychological evaluation can at times assist in finding the location of damage in the brain. This is referred to as localization of impair-ment. Many areas of the brain have been mapped with regard to the behavior or function associated with a particular region. This is particularly true for sensory input and motor output portions of the cerebral cortex. For example, the primary motor area, located in the posterior (the back end) of the frontal lobe, can be mapped for specific body part functions (e.g., hand, arm, foot, etc.). Parts of the brain and their associated functions will be discussed later in the physiology section.

The pattern of results from the evaluation can provide the neuropsy-chologist with the data to suggest a general location of tissue damage. For example, in some cases of traumatic brain injury, one side of the brain may be more affected than the other side. The localization of damage is of less importance for vocational planning, but may be more relevant for managing the client early in the process of rehabilitation. In cases where a neuropsy-chological evaluation is requested to determine if a client sustained a traumatic brain injury, it is more important to know the level and mechanism of impairment.

Treatment planning and monitoring of progress

The pattern of cognitive assets and deficits that is presented by a client can give the rehabilitation team valuable information about how best to provide treatment. If an individual presents with significant short-term verbal memory problems, but does well on tasks that require visual recall skills, treatment may be better focused upon compensating for verbal memory deficits by using visual cues and skills. In this situation, the client may be given a memory book in which to write down verbally presented information as a compensatory tool. Team members may be asked to show the client how to do a task, rather than merely telling the client what to do. We all have natural tendencies to recall information from verbal or visual cues, and this tendency may be altered by a traumatic brain injury. It is like being given directions to a location via a hand-drawn map or by writing down the street names and directions (e.g., turn left at 3rd Avenue, then make a right at Bertona Street). The neuropsychological evaluation is able to provide data that can be used to examine memory strengths and weaknesses. The neuropsychologist or other rehabilitation professional can then use this information to formulate an effective rehabilitation plan.

Monitoring client progress assists the neuropsychologist in understanding the process of recovery from brain injury. Repeating a battery or specific singular tests can provide information about changes in cognitive ability over time. This will be important in planning for job options. A person who improves little in a one-year time span is less likely to return to a work situation that approximates previous work tasks than a person who improves to a significant degree. This, however, is relative to the severity of the initial injury, as illustrated in Figure 2. The amount of change in this example is substantial over one year, yet this change can fall significantly short of the cognitive ability required for this client's previous job. If this person were to receive a third neuropsychological evaluation at two years post-injury, little change may have occurred. At that point, recovery may be slower and less noticeable on a day-to-day or month-to-month basis. The vocational counselor may then emphasize a different type of job focus requiring less cognitive complexity or involving tasks that are otherwise within the capability of the client.

In Figure 3, the client's progress in cognitive recovery is depicted as showing small improvements over the first year, yet that improvement is enough to approximate pre-injury cognitive skills required in a certain position. Vocational planning takes a different direction in this case, with emphasis upon building compensatory systems to allow the client to return to a previous work setting, with modifications.

Discharge planning

There may be certain everyday tasks for which a client must be considered capable before it is deemed safe for him to return home from an inpatient acute rehabilitation setting. An evaluation can provide input for discharge decisions involving the type of setting that is best for a client's discharge. Testing may suggest that it is unsafe for a client to live alone. The client may be unable to meet basic survival needs, and therefore, discharge to a

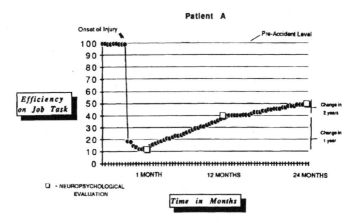

Figure 2 Change in cognitive function after a major decline of injury onset. Improvement after traumatic brain injury in this patient is gradual and linear, then slows by the end of the second year post-injury.

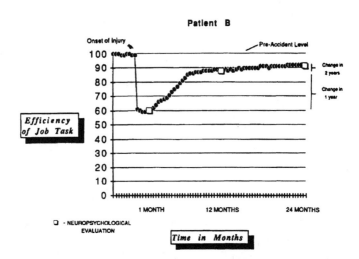

Figure 3 Change in cognitive function after a small decline at injury onset. Improvement in this patient is rapid within the first year and slows thereafter.

supervised living situation may be the most appropriate option. Other rehabilitation disciplines often provide further concrete data about a person's community safety (e.g., occupational therapy).

Community and everyday functioning

As noted above, the neuropsychological evaluation is important when determining the kind of setting and assistance that may be required for a client's return to the community. If a client with TBI has poor problem-solving skills, it may be necessary to closely monitor the person's checkbook balancing skills. If a person exhibits visual attention deficits, the client may need to be trained in community safety (e.g., crossing the street, or driving a car). The neuropsychological evaluation can provide assistance in clarifying issues of everyday functioning. Again, the relationship between test scores and everyday functioning has been referred to as the "ecological validity" of neuropsychological evaluation findings.

Vocational re-entry planning

Probably one of the most frequent uses of the neuropsychological evaluation is to assist in planning for employment or re-employment. In this regard, the evaluation provides valuable data in determining which jobs may be more suitable for a client to consider. The best fit between cognitive assets and deficits, behavioral functioning, interpersonal propensities, overlearned skills or old learning ability, and the specific job tasks is sought when making a job placement for a client with TBI. The evaluation, therefore, generates probability statements about which types of jobs are appropriate and which are not, narrowing the field of possibilities for the client based upon job task demands obtained from the vocational rehabilitation counselor.

It should be noted that there does not exist a one-to-one correspondence between neuropsychological data and job tasks. If this were the case, the process of matching a client with TBI to a job would be as simple as a computer match. Computer dating services operate on this principle, and this fact should speak for itself about how poor the match could be. The relationship between neuropsychological test scores and performance in daily life can be weak. This is why the evaluation includes more than just testing a client, but also involves gathering other relevant historical, medical, psychosocial, and vocational information.

Traditional psychological vs. neuropsychological evaluations

When a health care professional requests a neuropsychological evaluation, it is often helpful to specify exactly what one wishes to obtain. There is a difference between traditional psychological and neuropsychological evaluations. These distinctions are outlined below.

Psychological evaluation

Psychological assessment is primarily concerned with evaluating the emotional and behavioral status of the person in question. In this type of assessment, one is interested in knowing the psychological functioning of the individual. A psychological evaluation often consists of a review of medical records, a clinical interview with the client, sometimes an interview with a collateral source (e.g., a friend or family member), the administration of psychological tests, and the generation of a psychological report. Psychological tests assess a range of functioning: personality traits and interpersonal styles; mood status (presence and degree of depression, anger, or anxiety); nature and degree of psychopathology (psychotic thinking or long-standing inner conflicts); degree and nature of psychological stressors; marital satisfaction; dysfunctional irrational thinking; or personal coping styles, to name a few. Psychological tests come in the form of self-report inventories (e.g., Minnesota Multiphasic Personality Inventory, Beck Depression Inventory), clinician rating forms (e.g., Hamilton Rating Scale of Depression), and projective-type tests (e.g., Rorschach Inkblot Technique, Sentence Completion Test, and Thematic Apperception Test). The psychological report usually integrates all of the data gathered to yield a diagnosis, a case conceptualization of the relevant psychological variables, current stressors and conflicts, and in some cases a treatment plan.

At the end of psychological assessment report there often appears a diagnosis with associated codes taken from the *Diagnostic and Statistical Manual of Mental Disorders*, Fourth Edition.[13] This publication is a standard manual for coding all of the mental disorders. Please note that a psychological evaluation typically does not include tests to evaluate cognitive functioning. In some cases, a psychologist may administer a measure of global cognitive status such as a Mini-Mental State Examination.[14] This is a 30 total-points instrument in which the examiner asks the client questions about orientation (e.g., "Who is the president of the United States?"; "What day of the week is it?"), memory (e.g., asking the client to remember the names of three objects after five minutes elapsed time), and perceptual-motor ability (e.g., asking a client to draw a geometric figure). This type of mental status examination can detect the presence of significant or major cognitive impairment, such as in severe TBI or Alzheimer's Disease. It is less sensitive to more subtle problems.

Brief neuropsychological evaluation

There are some cases in which it may be too expensive or, for whatever reason, inappropriate to administer a full battery of neuropsychological tests. A brief neuropsychological evaluation will include a review of records, clinical interview with the client and a collateral person or significant other, and the administration of selected cognitive tests (e.g., the Wechsler Adult Intelligence Scale – III given with a memory measure such as the Wechsler Memory Scale – III). Some psychologists will also add psychological tests to augment the cognitive data (e.g., MMPI-2) or brief measures of academic ability. A report is generated from the above data. This brief evaluation can often answer a number of questions such as the following:

1. Does this client have cognitive impairment and is there evidence of brain dysfunction or disease?

2. Do the test results suggest the need for a comprehensive neuropsychological evaluation?
3. What is the level of this person's intellectual functioning and can the person carry out certain job tasks?
4. Does this client have attention and concentration problems that warrant further assessment?
5. Does this client have the potential to benefit from cognitive compensatory training?
6. How well does this person read?
7. How well does this person write?
8. What level of arithmetic can this person perform consistently?
9. Does this client's visual ability require further assessment?
10. Does this client's emotional status contribute significantly to his or her cognitive performance? Is treatment necessary for the emotional component?

These are but a few of the questions that can be answered with a brief neuropsychological evaluation. More complex questions may be answered with a comprehensive evaluation and are discussed later in this chapter. Some psychologists may say that they are conducting neuropsychological testing, but in reality they are doing brief neuropsychological evaluations. The position taken here is that outside of the questions mentioned above, the brief neuropsychological evaluation falls short of yielding comprehensive data that are important to vocational planning or defining in a more precise way what is needed by a particular client. In the same way that you shop for a new car, the rehabilitation professional should be an informed consumer about the product that is being purchased.

Comprehensive neuropsychological evaluation

In this type of evaluation, a full range of tests is administered, depending upon the orientation of the neuropsychologist who is conducting the evaluation. A review of records, a clinical interview with client and collateral resources, the administration of neuropsychological and psychological tests, and the generation of an often lengthy report are the main components of a comprehensive neuropsychological evaluation. The testing time alone will often require a full day.

Cost

In general, the old adage "You get what you pay for" applies well to neuropsychological evaluations. Such evaluations are not standardized as to cost. Costs can relate to a number of variables, such as the experience of the neuropsychologist, the number of tests administered, the geographic location of the neuropsychologist, the particular orientation of the neuropsychologist, whether or not a psychometrist administers the test, whether or not a feedback session is built into the total fee, and a host of other factors. An estimation of the range of costs for a comprehensive evaluation that includes the administration of all tests and the generation of a report without the cost of a client feedback session is currently between $1000 to $1,500 (1998). Some neuropsychologists, particularly in forensic cases, will charge several thousand dollars more. To some degree, this can be due to extensive records review. On the other hand, paying $1,500 for a neuropsychological evaluation does not guarantee a quality report according to the standards of the person referring an individual for evaluation. One may also not be guaranteed that specific referral questions will be answered. Bear in mind that this is a free enterprise system and if you are the consumer (if you are purchasing an evaluation for a client), it is always important to approach the purchase of neuropsychological services as one would approach the purchase of other services.

Requesting a rehabilitation-oriented report

As mentioned above, it is important to expect that you will generally pay a fair amount for a comprehensive neuropsychological evaluation. The rehabilitation counselor is likely to invest a great deal of time in a particular client, and the neuropsychological evaluation can yield much in the way of rehabilitation direction and benefit. For this to happen, it is vitally important that the vocational rehabilitation counselor or other health care professional be assertive in obtaining the information that will answer particular rehabilitation questions. The following then are general guidelines that can be of assistance in formulating evaluation requests:

1. List the problems or obstacles in the case. Before requesting an evaluation, list all of the client's problems and obstacles that prevent this person from obtaining and/or maintaining a job. This will help generate the questions that are to be asked in the evaluation. Think of any remaining gaps in the data to account for a problem (e.g., "Why is it that the client is always late for job interviews?").
2. Brainstorm a list of questions to be answered by an evaluation. This point will be discussed further; however, suffice it to say that a listing of questions will help better conceptualize the case. Some critical questions may not require a neuropsychologist, but rather a speech and language pathologist, or an occupational therapist for an answer.
3. Keep questions rehabilitation-oriented or functional. It is less helpful for a vocational counselor to find out between which fissures of the cerebral cortex and at what lesion depth a client's contusion reaches than a person's specific cognitive assets and deficits at a particular point in time. You may wish to know what residual assets remain after a traumatic brain injury upon which rehabilitation can capitalize. It can often be expedient to build a vocational rehabilitation plan upon residual cognitive assets. You may want to know what type of compensatory approach will work best with a particular client to help

make decisions about what other services are needed. It may also be important to know whether or not to expect further cognitive improvement in time to best target the appropriate work goal. These are examples of more rehabilitation-oriented questions.
4. Be persistent in finding out the information needed from the neuropsychologist. The evaluation generates a plethora of data. Such evaluations are often conducted in the context of an even larger comprehensive assessment of the client, such as in a brain injury rehabilitation program. Therefore, the neuropsychologist may have access to data beyond the tests themselves. The combination of neuropsychological testing data and, for example, the client's performance on an everyday task (e.g., budgeting) done in occupational therapy may have implications for work access. It may be important to pursue such valuable information from the neuropsychologist.

Physiology

An in-depth discussion of brain physiology is beyond the scope of this chapter. The physiology of the major brain structures that is relevant to traumatic brain injury will be presented.

Although the brain has been studied for many centuries, only within the past 50 years have we learned more about the relationship between physiology and behavior. In this regard, the medical field is still at an early stage in its understanding of brain functioning. We are now able to understand the structure of the brain yet we are still short on information regarding what each part of the brain is responsible for the complexities of intra- and inter-component functioning.

David H. Hubel,[15] Professor of Neurobiology at Harvard Medical School, has noted the following:

> The brain is a tissue. It is a complicated, intricately woven tissue, like nothing else we know of in the universe, but it is composed of cells as any tissue is. They are, to be sure, highly specialized cells, but they function according to the laws that govern any other cells. Their electrical and chemical signals can be detected, recorded, and interpreted, and their chemicals can be identified; the connections that constitute the brain's woven felt work can be mapped. In short, the brain can be studied, just as the kidney can. The problem comes when we ask about understanding, because such a word carries with it the implication of a sudden revelation or dawning. The existence of a moment when we might be said to leave the darkness of the tunnel. It is not clear to me that there can be such a moment, or that we will know when it comes (p. 3).

In short, despite the rapid growth in knowledge in the neurosciences, a clear understanding of how the brain works remains largely a mystery. By understanding brain–behavior relationships from the combined views of neuroscientists, neurologists, neuropsychologists, and other allied health professionals, we may better understand, and hopefully predict and correct brain problems.

Major brain structures relevant to traumatic brain injury

Covered here are the three major areas of the brain that can become damaged in traumatic brain injury. The brain itself is a gel-type mass that sits in a bath of water within the skull. If one were to remove the brain from the skull, one would see a gray, convoluted mass that is much akin to the consistency of very thick pasta. The gray outer surface of the brain comprises the cerebral cortex. It is relatively thin, consisting of five or six layers of cells, and is frequently referred to as the *gray matter*. Directly beneath the cortex lies an intricate system of conducting fibers, often referred to as the *white matter*. These fibers provide communicating links between different areas of the brain.

The brain is comprised of two roughly symmetrical halves, or hemispheres. These hemispheres are connected by a very thick bundle of nerves (white matter) called the *corpus collosum* (Latin for *large body*). The corpus collosum is the main communication pathway between the two hemispheres. Structurally, the two hemispheres are not exactly symmetrical. For example, the right parietal lobe consists of a greater portion of space than the left parietal lobe when examined from the interior portion of the brain. This inner brain structure allows for communication between the two hemispheres. Each hemisphere of the brain can be mapped out into four regions or lobes (Figure 4). These lobes are not distinct structures in and of themselves. Just as imaginary lines as represented on a map dividing parts of the city, the lobes of the brain roughly correspond to specific areas of a hemisphere. The brain works as a whole, and the whole is generally believed to be a greater functional entity than the sum of its individual parts. This is likely true for brain functioning, because any particular action results from the mass effect of a number of different parts and connections.

Frontal lobes

The frontal lobes are probably the area of the brain that most differentiates humans from lower animal forms. Certainly the frontal lobes are much more developed in humans than in animals; the area of the human brain that is represented by the frontal lobes is greater than any other animal form. The frontal lobes are responsible for integrating many of the other functions of the brain. The term *executive function* has been associated with the frontal lobe system. Just as a business executive needs to organize many people and pieces of information, and plan ahead, the frontal lobes are responsible for

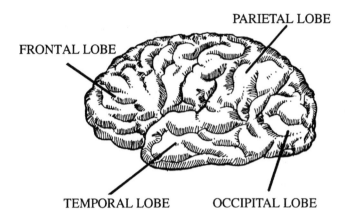

FRONTAL LOBE

PARIETAL LOBE

TEMPORAL LOBE

OCCIPITAL LOBE

Figure 4 The four major lobes of the cerebral cortex.

similar kinds of functions in everyday behavior. They are largely responsible for complex thinking, the ability to anticipate and plan, initiate action, and execute sequences of behavior. The frontal lobes are also responsible for aspects of personality and the regulation of emotions. The system that connects the frontal lobes with the inner brain structures of the limbic system is involved in emotional expression and regulation. Some scientists believe that this part of the brain is also essential for self-awareness and the ability to observe and correct one's own behavior. Because the frontal lobes have an integrating function, they have numerous connections to other parts of the brain. For example, to be self-aware of one's own conversation skills, a person needs to integrate visual information, auditory perception, verbal output, be able to articulate and search for correct words, use abstract thinking to track humor or other complex information, as well as recall and store things people may have said during a conversation. All of these may need to be put together or integrated by the frontal lobes.

Temporal lobes

The temporal lobes are thought to have a major role in memory, particularly short-term or what is called recent memory. Memory is a complex phenomenon. It can include storage of old information (e.g., your place of birth, the alphabet, recalling the face of that tyrannical teacher who put you in the corner in second grade) as well as newly learned information, which is called short-term memory (e.g., remembering what you had for breakfast this morning). The left temporal lobe is thought to emphasize verbal information, whereas the right temporal lobe is more responsible for the storage of visual information. For example, if one were to recall the information written in this chapter, it is likely that both the left and right temporal lobes are involved. This is due to the fact that this text's print constitutes both visual and language stimuli. The temporal lobe is also important for perceiving auditory information in sequencing input. As will be noted later, the frontal and temporal lobes play major roles in traumatic brain injury. The connection of the temporal lobes to inner limbic structures, and specifically the hippocampus, is thought to be the system associated with what has been termed *working memory*. Working memory is that initial and small storage area that allows processing of ongoing events and cognitive procedures. Most tasks of everyday functioning involve an aspect of working memory abilities.

Parietal lobes

The parietal lobes are important for visual-spatial organizational ability. This part of the brain assists in interpreting information that is delivered through the visual senses, and is known as spatial ability. For most people, the right parietal lobe is more responsible for analyzing and organizing spatial information. For example, a mechanic may employ visual organizational skills in assembling and figuring out problems with a carburetor. Awareness of three-dimensional objects and designs, and the ability to integrate motor activities (e.g., drawing an object on a piece of paper by looking at the object) is a function of this part of the brain. It is thought that the left parietal lobe is important for executing arithmetic problems, comprehending and repeating speech, and reading and writing abilities.

Occipital lobes

The occipital lobes are located in the rear portion of the brain. They are responsible for visual perception, interpreting and recognizing visual sense input. For example, the primary visual cortex, which is in the very rear portion of the occipital lobes, receives direct input from the retina, through a specific visual nerve pathway. The stimuli that enter through the retina of the eyes are projected back to the occipital lobes. This information must then be interpreted, a process which is called perception. These lobes are also responsible for recognizing and interpreting size and shape dimensions of visual input.

Limbic system

Beneath the cerebral cortex lie other brain structures that are relevant to this discussion of brain physiology in traumatic brain injury. Immediately underneath the cortex is an important structure known as the limbic system (Figure 5). This system is connected to the brain stem, which will be discussed later. There are a number of specific structures that make up the limbic system including the amygdala, hippocampus, basal ganglia, septum, fornix, cingulate gyrus, and parts of the anterior thalamus, and the hypothalamus. The limbic system is considered a deeper brain structure and may be considered a more primitive part of the brain from an evolutionary perspective. This is

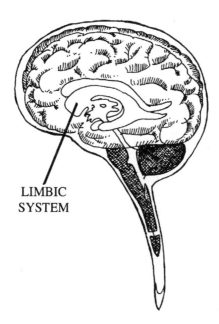

LIMBIC
SYSTEM

Figure 5 The limbic system.

because the limbic system appears to be similar in all mammals. This system is essential for regulating emotion, initially storing and manipulating information, and distributing information to recent verbal and visual memory. It is also responsible for different components of body movements. It is termed a *system* because the structures of the limbic system work as a whole with higher level cortical structures in a highly interconnected way.

Human behaviors, such as emotions, are a result of a stream of events in the limbic system. These events are not things we think about, but rather they occur in microseconds throughout the day. For example, if one were walking in the house and somebody suddenly jumped out of a closet, there would be an immediate fear response and a rush of emotions that likely occur without cognition. Reflexive motor responses would occur, along with an instant change in hormonal balance. Heart rate, breathing rate, and blood pressure may be immediately altered. Cognitions about fear might follow quickly after the event.

Aggressive and fear reactions are mediated by the limbic system. Since there is a physical reaction to such things as fear, there are connections to other parts of the nervous system, for example, which control heart rate, respiration, blood pressure, and perspiration. Any of these functions can be altered in traumatic brain injury due to damage to the limbic system. Limbic system damage may occur directly as a result of the physics of traumatic brain injury, but the system may also malfunction because of disconnections to the limbic areas themselves.

Brain stem

Lying beneath the limbic system is the brain stem. This may be considered the base of the brain. Below it extends the spinal cord. The brain stem contains other significant structures including the reticular formation, pons, medulla oblongata, substantia nigra, and the cerebellum. The brain stem plays an important role in such basic functions as heart rate, rhythmic breathing, and the sleep–wake cycle. A system known as the reticular activating system is essential in regulating sleep and alertness. For example, while sleeping, most of us are unaware of small noises or normal sounds that occur during the night. However, if there is an unidentified sound or some unusual occurrence, the reticular activating system responds by awakening the person. The system acts as an ongoing security monitor for events that are intentionally not paid attention to, particularly in the sleeping state. Damage to the brain stem can result in problems with sleep cycles and alertness, loss of consciousness, coma, or fluctuation in alertness and attention. The brain stem can be damaged since the physical forces of an injury can result in the brain rotating on the brain stem, causing contusions, bruises, or other problems in the brain stem.

Mechanisms of traumatic brain injury

There are various ways in which the brain can become injured in a traumatic event. Traumatic brain injury will be differentiated from other forms of brain problems such as aneurysms, arteriovenous malformations, brain tumor problems, and cerebral vascular accidents (CVAs, also known as stroke). Traumatic brain injury occurs often as a result of two major forces (see Figure 6). In an

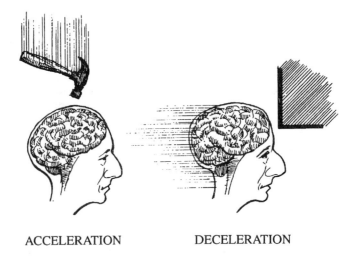

ACCELERATION   DECELERATION

Figure 6 Mechanisms of traumatic brain injury. Motor vehicle accidents, falls, and similar types of injuries in brain damage, often due to acceleration and/or deceleration types of impacts.

acceleration injury, a moving object strikes a stationary head. For example, a construction worker may be standing below a building and scaffolding may fall on this person's head. In a *deceleration* injury, a moving head strikes a stationary object. This often occurs in motor vehicle accidents in which the head and body are brought to an abrupt halt by striking a stationary object, such as a guardrail, windshield, or wall. Another example of a deceleration injury is when a bicyclist falls and strikes the ground. In many motor vehicle accidents, which are the cause of close to one-half of all traumatic brain injuries, there is often a combination of acceleration and deceleration forces that account for damage that occurs to the brain.

There is a distinction between an *open head injury* and a *closed head injury*. In the former, an object penetrates the skull resulting in brain damage. For example, in a skull fracture injury, part of the skull may be depressed into the brain resulting in damage. In closed head injury, the brain may be damaged within the skull due to acceleration or deceleration forces. Damage in the brain can be considered diffuse (i.e., spread throughout the brain), or more localized (in specific areas of the brain). It is more often the case in traumatic brain injury that there is a combination of both diffuse and localized damage.

Damage can present as *brain contusions*, which are bruises on the brain, much akin to bruises received on other parts of the body. (A contusion causes tissue damage and bleeding.) If a contusion is on the cerebral cortex, it is referred to as a cerebral contusion. If the bruising occurs in the brain stem area, it would be called a brain stem contusion. Damage to the brain can also occur as a result of a hematoma. A *hematoma* is a collection of blood in a certain confined space in the brain.

Another mechanism of TBI is what is called *diffuse axonal injury*. This occurs when the axons (which comprise part of a neuron) in the cortex are damaged, often globally, across the cortex. Axons tend to be thick, interconnected, and healthy. After brain injury, these axons may be stretched, sheared, and torn. In some cases, the axons may be intact, but do not conduct electrical impulses as well or at all. Diffuse axonal injury can result in cognitive and emotional impairments of many different sorts.

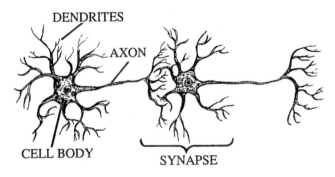

Figure 7 The neuron including the axon, dendrites, and synapse.

Common areas of damage: frontal and temporal lobes

There are areas in the brain that are more vulnerable to damage from the physical forces that occur in traumatic brain injury. As depicted in Figure 8, the frontal and temporal lobes are more frequently involved in such injuries.

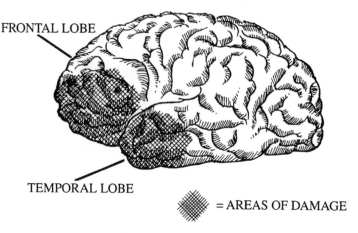

Figure 8   Common areas of damage after traumatic brain injury. The shaded areas represent the most vulnerable areas of damage. These include hematomas, contusions, and cerebral hemorrhages.

The brain is not uniformly shaped and fits rather snugly into the skull. It is important to notice where the temporal and frontal lobes lie. They rest on bony structures inside the skull. Figure 9 shows a view of the base of the skull from above. Neurological studies in which computed axial tomographies (CAT scans) have been obtained on clients with traumatic brain injury consistently show damage (contusions, hematomas) in the frontal and temporal regions. This is because they are easily damaged by the bony ridges and protrusions which characterize the skull in these areas. The part of the skull that corresponds to the occipital lobe (in the rear portion of the brain) does not have these bony ridges and tends to be smooth. Fewer primary problems are seen in that region of the brain in TBI. Frontal lobe damage is frequently associated with changes in personality, behavior problems (e.g., agitation, anger outbursts, or inappropriate social behavior); problems with executive functions (complex problem-solving, the ability to deal with multiple inputs, sequencing events, abstract thinking, creativity, and novel approaches to problem situations); and a general decrease in adaptive functioning in everyday situations. Memory deficits also are cardinal features of TBI and relate to temporal lobe damage.

As was mentioned previously, damage to the brain can occur by blows to the head from any angle or location. Examples are *coup* and *contrecoup* injuries. Coup (the French word for "blow" or "strike") injuries are the direct

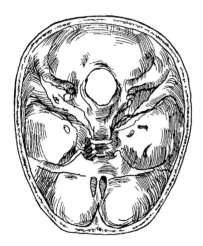

Figure 9 Bony ridges of the skull as seen from the top view. The frontal and temporal lobes rest on these ridges, making them vulnerable to damage when a sufficient force is applied to the head.

result of a blow to the head. Contrecoup (French for "opposite the blow") injuries occur when the head is struck at one point, and the brain is damaged at another point by rebounding off the inside of the skull. In some cases the brain damage may not occur directly opposite the point of impact, due to the fact that the brain can move around inside the skull. In penetrating head traumas, such as bullet or shrapnel wounds, the object that penetrates the skull may deflect off structures inside the brain/skull, and exit the skull at a point other than opposite the entry site. Damage can be just as diffuse and widespread as in a closed head injury, or may be quite localized.

The brain is fully supplied by blood and oxygen. To get blood and oxygen to brain tissue, a complex system of arteries is needed. Unfortunately, this affords much opportunity in brain injury for contusions and hematomas to occur and cause tissue damage since the brain contains so many arteries and blood vessels. In the case of a hematoma, a collection of blood can occur in several spaces in the brain resulting in brain tissue being compressed and, therefore, damaged in that area. When this happens to a great extent, surgery may be required to evacuate this hematoma. A collection of blood in the brain can result in increased pressure inside of the brain. This is called increased *intracranial pressure* (ICP). Intracranial pressure can also increase due to swelling of brain tissue. This is caused by increased blood volume going to the brain. As is true in other body tissues, swelling occurs in the area of injury. In the brain, this is referred to as brain edema. Many of these types of problems are treated in the trauma unit, emergency room, or intensive care unit. Such difficulties may further be treated while on a neurosurgery or neurology unit or in an acute hospitalization phase. Once medically stable, the client may be transferred to the first phase of rehabilitation.

Linkages between cognitive functioning and behavioral impairments

Any discussion of the cognitive consequences of traumatic brain injury cannot be made in isolation from the total clinical picture presented by TBI clients. Many aspects of these clients' lives are affected. Unfortunately, many of these affected areas interact with each other. Each area should be addressed by comprehensive rehabilitation efforts. The success of treatment can often be contingent upon how the client is functioning in other aspects of life.

Interplay between cognition and behavior disorders

It is common after traumatic brain injury that cognitive deficits are accompanied by behavioral disturbances. An individual may have both problem-solving and memory impairments, as well as problems with anger and depression. The combination of these cognitive behavioral problems can wreak havoc if one tries to return such an individual to work too quickly and without proper rehabilitation. If one simply targets the memory problem and does not deal with the anger or depression, problems will likely remain in trying to re-employ this individual. What follows are some of the behavioral disturbances that occur after traumatic brain injury which may need to be addressed through the process of rehabilitation.

Problematic behaviors

There are basically two major categories of behavioral disturbances. **Disinhibition** refers to the process of losing inhibitory controls over action and emotions. The client may or may not be aware of a change in his ability to inhibit responses, such as anger outbursts. Most of us, for example, would be able to inhibit tomato-throwing behavior if standing in a five-item or less grocery line and the first person in line has a cart full of 30 items and is paying by check. Usually, those without brain injury are able to inhibit these impulses. After traumatic brain damage, disinhibition means that tomato-throwing behavior and other impulsive displays might not be suppressed even though the person may wish to do so or is unaware that this is inappropriate. There are a number of disinhibition problems that cover aggression, inappropriate social, verbal, or sexual behavior, and amount of emotional output (see Table 1).

Another type of behavioral disturbance involves difficulty initiating action. **Initiation deficits** refer to the absence of action or emotion, or an absence of spontaneous behavior and initiative. For example, an individual may be trained to carry out a single task, but may not initiate the next task or action. This individual would then need periodic and consistent cueing in order to complete a job task. Behavioral deficits tend to come in the forms as noted in Table 1.

Table 1   A Typology of Affective and Behavioral Disturbances
After Brain Injury

Behavioral symptom	Description
Inappropriate abrupt action	The person responds to a situation too quickly and without thinking about the adequacy or consequences of the behavior; characterized by doing before thinking.
Tangential verbal output	Expresses one thought after another in disconnected or unrelated sequences; observed as rambling speech, or the person is unable to get to the point.
Excessive verbal output	Provides too much information; content may be overly detailed or redundant; may be unaware of conversation turn exchange signals, or unable to terminate conversation; seen as excessively talkative.
Verbal interruptions	Inserts comments that disrupt the flow of conversation or the task at hand; may force other person to relinquish conversational turn before completing a thought.
Inappropriate topic selection	Poor discrimination of appropriate topics for the social context. Revealing statements about personal matters, relationships, mood, and feelings that are inappropriate for the social context or level of relationship; excessive self-disclosure.
Inappropriate word choice	Use of profanity or emotionally charged words that are inappropriate for the social context. Overly explicit descriptions and explanations.
Physical proximity violation	Positions body within spatial proximity of another person that is inappropriate for the level of relationship or social context; person is seen as violating personal space margins; physical touch without sexual intent.
Sexual inappropriateness	Acts with the intent of developing an intimate or sexual contact that is inappropriate for the level of relationship or is in violation of social mores (e.g., an adult with an adolescent minor); conversation contains sexual innuendo or lewd comments. May interpret others' expression of friendship as sexual advances, and respond as noted above.
Poor social judgment	Unaware of, or does not apply rules governing social behavior to one's own situation; does not consider personal safety or safety of others in a social context; may be viewed as rude, immature, coarse, or showing minimal social tact. Violates rules of etiquette (but not as a result of cognitive deficits in judgment).

Table 1 (continued)   A Typology of Affective and Behavioral Disturbances
                          After Brain Injury

Behavioral symptom	Description
Irritability	Feelings of annoyance or impatience; may accompany restlessness; easily provoked but generally does not escalate into an anger outburst. Tends to be a constant state, usually neither improving nor worsening by a significant degree; may be seen by others as grouchy, grumpy, or pouting.
Lability of affect	Magnitude of affect displayed is disproportionate to the antecedent event or social context and does not necessarily reflect the true nature, extent, or feelings.
Anxious affect and rumination	Feelings of worry, tension, fear, uncertainty about the future. Complains or verbalizes concern over trivia.
Anger transition/verbal	An escalation of verbal output, where pitch, volume, and/or speaking rate increase, dysfluency occurs, aggressive content is delivered. The person's behavior falls within socially appropriate realms. A building-up phase toward an angry outburst occurs.
Anger transition/behavioral	Facial flush, posture is threatening, personal space may be violated, body positions are exaggerated, agitated behavior is evident (e.g., hair pulling, wringing of hands, clutching of the fist).
Anger outburst/verbal	Explosive speech, screaming, abusive language, forceful or harmful content, self-deprecating content, or threats toward another person occur.
Anger outburst/behavioral	Hitting objects, striking out at individuals or objects, exaggerated motions of arms and hands, forceful or destructive actions occur.
Absence or decrease in self-directed action	Decrease in spontaneous behaviors emitted by the person is evidenced. Requires prompts for the person to initiate action.
Dysphoric mood	Downcast facial expression, tearfulness, verbalizations of sadness, hopelessness, helplessness, low self-esteem; paucity of interest in pleasant events is demonstrated.
Restricted, flat or blunted affect	Display of affect is less than proportionate to the event; face can be expressionless, voice monotonous, movement and facial expression may fail to reflect stated feelings.

Evidence of these behavioral problems is not present in each client with brain injury, and it is difficult to predict a prognosis for these difficulties. To assess behavioral disturbances, it is often helpful to interview many sources. A family report and the client's self-report are often useful to obtain, particularly to compare similarities and differences in perception between client and family member. Clinician and staff observations provide information that can be compared with that from home or work environment settings. A comparison can be made between a person's behavior in a structured setting (e.g., in a clinic or on a job tryout or station) vs. a community setting (e.g., in a job interview, interacting with co-workers, or working alone without supervision). Once behavior problems are adequately assessed and defined, training problems and strategies can then be developed and executed.

Sequences of behaviors

Another important aspect of the interplay between cognitive and behavior difficulties is the sequence of events that can occur under stressful conditions. Figure 10 depicts components that can be involved in a person's poor performance on a job task.

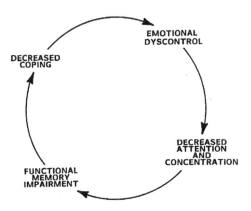

Figure 10 Sequences of behavior after traumatic brain injury. This cycle can explain how a downward spiral of daily dysfunction can occur as a function of problems at any point along the cycle.

Poor performance at the work site, home, or in the community can result from problems at any point in this cycle. Decreased attention can lead to poor memory ability that creates a situation where the individual loses coping ability. This may increase anger or depression that then leads to further attention deficits and so forth. Such vicious cycles are often prompted by minor frustrations or obstacles that may occur at a work site or in other community or family settings. Effective intervention is directed at any or all components in the sequence. When analyzing job performance, it is important to find at which point in the task sequence the client fails. Interventions can then be better designed and implemented.

Implications for vocational planning

Given the interplay between cognitive and behavioral variables, it makes sense to obtain a thorough assessment of all these variables. A neuropsychological assessment can cover most of the cognitive variables, whereas input from a behavioral specialist (usually a person with a master's degree in applied behavior analysis) or a good behavioral, clinical, or counseling psychologist can assist in evaluating behavioral disturbance. Some employers may be worried about an adult with brain injury who may have had some anger difficulties since the onset of injury. It would be important to look at this client's history before and after injury for indications of verbal or physical aggressiveness. Past history continues to be the best predictor of future behavior. If one was prone to anger outbursts before brain injury, it is likely that this person would also have anger dyscontrol after brain injury. There are fewer cases in which a person was aggressive before brain injury and afterward became more docile. Therefore, if employers are concerned about an individual's behavioral disturbances on the job, it is prudent to obtain a thorough history of behavioral problems since the onset of traumatic brain injury. Behavioral disorders should not necessarily preclude an individual from desired employment. Much of the behavior management literature would suggest that many of these difficulties, as noted in Table 1, can be remediated or at least controlled to the point of being less of an issue on the job. Such individuals may reveal their behavioral disturbances in the home environment while maintaining their composure on the job.

Often clients can be taught self-management skills and also ways to monitor their behavior on the job site. In situations where the behavior problem is difficult to control, pharmacological help can augment behavioral training benefits. Pharmacological agents such as buspirone, a longer acting anxiolytic, can be beneficial to the client without oversedation. The longer the behavioral problem has been in existence and the more severe the traumatic brain injury, the more difficult such problems are to remediate. A comprehensive assessment will likely work best to thoroughly evaluate the range of cognitive and behavioral deficits that may pose barriers to successful work access or reemployment.

Generalizing learned skills from the clinic and work trial to the actual job situation will be the trickiest part of rehabilitation. Clients with cognitive deficits have, by definition, decreased ability to transfer learning from one situation to the next. Simulating as closely as possible the actual work situation through a job station or work trial can be helpful in vocational planning. It would also be helpful to evaluate the job for high-risk situations that may lead to behavioral problems. For example, if the work situation is noisy and there are many interruptions and distractions, the client may become frustrated and, consequently, angry. In addition, an individual's concentration can be interrupted and productivity may drop. One may also want to test the limits in a work trial situation to evaluate at what point cognitive and behavioral problems interfere with job performance. This is always done with the client's permission. Testing the limits will also better prepare you to anticipate problems that may occur on the job itself. More specific rehabilitation therapies can then be implemented to overcome some of the more frequent barriers that may emerge to testing the limits.

Functional areas of cognition in neuropsychological assessment

There are several major areas of cognitive functioning that are assessed through a neuropsychological evaluation. They are not necessarily distinct, and there is frequently overlap between areas that are assessed by different neuropsychological tests. Most reports will be broken down into subsections such as in the outline presented below. Other reports will have each of the areas covered within the body of the report but not broken down by sections. In other cases, individual neuropsychologists may interpret a test result to reflect a particular area of cognitive functioning while other neuropsychologists may interpret it within a different area. This will naturally become confusing, and you may need to clarify particular results with the neuropsychologist with whom you are working. One framework for reviewing the different areas of cognition is presented below.

General neuropsychological functioning

The concept

In any assessment a global estimate of the client's general cognitive level is desired. A global index of general neuropsychological functioning can assist in determining the amount of presumed decline after injury. Further, a global index of functioning assists in generating predictions about long-term vocational outcome. Because a measure of general functioning covers a wide range of abilities, it often cannot yield any specific information about a client with specific assets and deficits. In essence, such an index is an average in much the same way that a bowling average summarizes one's game. This bowling average does not give information about individual game scores, but does help determine handicaps to apply to certain bowlers.

From such a global estimate of neuropsychological functioning, judgements can be made as to the relative position of each individual test score. A measure of this type is the Halstead Impairment Index, which is based on the Halstead Reitan Neuropsychological Battery. The original battery consists of seven indexed tests in which the number of tests scored in the impaired range (based on cutoff scores) determines the level of general impairment. The scores range from 0.0 (normal range) to 1.0 (severe impairment). A recent expansion of the Impairment Index is the Neuropsychological Deficit Scale. This scale combines cutoff scores from several other tests and procedures from the battery to yield a total score. Many neuropsychologists also use the Full Scale I.Q. score from the Wechsler Adult Intelligence Scale (WAIS-R, WAIS-III) as a measure of general level of functioning. The neuropsychologist usually calculates or estimates a client's pre-injury general intellectual functioning based on age, education, and occupational background as noted earlier in this chapter. This estimate is compared to the index of general neuropsychological functioning to determine if change had occurred as a result of injury. Some of the more common indices of general functioning are listed in Appendix B.

Vocational implications

1. General neuropsychological functioning can assist with examining long-term vocational potential. The degree to which the person approximates premorbid or pre-injury cognitive functioning can offer a rough estimate of the degree to which the person will be able to approach pre-injury job tasks.
2. Indices that were mentioned above should not be regarded as absolute values because specific areas of functioning must be examined before making any decisions about work trials or job placement. A person may test as having general functioning equivalent to estimated premorbid levels, but have specific new deficits that may greatly interfere with pre-injury tasks.
3. In examining indices of general functioning, examine impaired test scores to see if client's performances are far beyond or close to the cutoff scores for brain impairment. In both situations the person may have a high impairment index yet present with a totally different clinical picture – these impairment indices do not have a range.

Sensory motor integrity

The concept
A distinction needs to be made between damage that occurs in the central nervous system (i.e., the brain and spinal column) vs. injuries to the body peripheral to the central nervous system. Such peripheral injuries can include fractures to the bones in the hand or nerve damage in the arm that would result in fine-motor dexterity problems. Neuropsychological assessment will not distinguish between what is brain-related vs. peripheral impairment. On a functional basis, however, it will give information about what a person can and cannot do regardless of cause. After traumatic brain injury, problems can also occur in sensory and motor segments of the brain. Motor and sensory functions are contralateralized; that is, the left hemisphere of the brain operates the right side of the body, and the right hemisphere of the

brain operates the left side of the body. Motor speed and strength can be lessened as a result of brain injury. Sensations such as pressure, temperature, and pain can be affected, for example, in the hands, fingertips, arms, and legs. A traumatic brain injury, especially a severe one, will generally affect several areas of life function.

Vocational implications

1. Sensory-motor functioning can make a difference for individuals who rely upon their hands for their trade. Electronics assemblers, mechanics, carpenters, and people in other professions that require both gross-motor and fine-motor abilities may be affected by changes in this area. Particular attention to a job task and its requirements for hand functioning should be made and discussed with the neuropsychologist. In some cases, a more refined assessment of hand function by an occupational therapist may be needed. Information from the physical therapist and the physiatrist should also be obtained to gain a full assessment of a client's motor functioning.
2. The neuropsychological evaluation does not routinely cover balance and gait sensory-motor functions. The physical therapist and physiatrist need to be consulted for this information as it relates to job tasks.
3. Speed, strength, and accuracy data are often needed to make determinations about the best fit between the client and the job. A person may have good strength and dexterity, but have motor slowing that results in poor productivity (e.g., on an assembly line).
4. A client's performance in a work trial situation may need to be observed carefully to see if any failures are due to sensory-motor difficulties vs. visual-perceptual problems. For example, a person may be able to execute a task manually, but may not have the visual or perceptual skills (i.e., analyzing the visual information correctly) to carry out the task.

Attention and concentration

The concept

Assuming that a client's sensory-motor functioning is within normal limits, the next level of analysis is in the area of attention and concentration. To carry out most cognitive tasks, a basic requirement is to attend and to sustain concentration on that task. If a client is required to listen to customers by telephone and that person's attentional abilities are poor, the client may not be able to remember requests or employ problem-solving strategies to help a customer. Most job tasks will require some form of visual and/or auditory/verbal attention ability. A diamond cutter or electronic assembler spends much work time concentrating on visual details and coordinating (hand) responses with what they see before them. These two professions require a large amount of fine-motor dexterity along with excellent visual attention abilities. A switchboard operator likely expends much mental energy on auditory/verbal attention in listening to people all day. Any type of counselor also uses verbal attention abilities daily. In most work settings, it is important for the employee to focus attention on the task at hand and block out distractions (e.g., other people talking, visual commotion in the work area, and noise). Employees often need to use visual and auditory attention, but they must also focus their attention (concentrate) and be able to be free from distractions. After traumatic brain injury, attention and concentration deficits are common. This can be a major obstacle to successful re-employment.

Vocational implications

1. It is easy to take for granted the amount of attention and concentration that is required of certain job tasks. Careful examination of potential job placements and settings will be important for traumatically brain-injured clients. These problems occur very frequently within this population and, therefore, planning for maximizing performance through minimizing job-site distractions would be helpful.
2. Attention and concentration are separate entities. Careful examination of the type of basic attentional difficulties that the client may have will help in making job-setting modifications that facilitate attention and the capacity to maintain focus (concentrate).
3. The client with a TBI can be taught ways to maximize attentional skills. Self-management techniques may help the client focus on a task. Anxiety and irritability can contribute to attentional difficulties and you may need to have clients assessed relative to managing these concerns if the techniques being taught are not helpful.
4. Physical problems, such as pain, fatigue, and sleep problems can also greatly contribute to attentional deficits. Establishing a client's best functional hours of the day may initially assist you in better programming the client's work schedule. Building the client's physical and mental tolerance to the work situation can also help.
5. Modifying the work environment may be essential for the survivor with a brain injury. Having the individual work alone, with minimal telephone or in-person distractions may work better, at least initially.

Recent verbal and visual-spatial memory

The concept

Memory is multifaceted in nature. Although you may hear people talking about having a good vs. a poor memory, it is more accurate to say that people have particular assets and deficits in their memory capabilities. These capacities are not to be confused with the previously discussed attention and concentration abilities that are important underpinnings to memory functioning. There is also a difference between long-term and short-term memory.

As mentioned earlier, it is the short-term memory that is most affected by brain impairment. As traumatic brain injury becomes severe, however, long-term memory can also be a problem. For example, a 25-year-old male client of the author was involved in a bicycle vs. car accident and sustained a very severe closed head injury. He was a Ph.D. candidate in engineering at the time of his accident. After emerging from coma and stabilizing medically, the client was followed in outpatient rehabilitation. Almost nine months after the injury, he still could not remember whether he had obtained a master's degree or was in a Ph.D. program. This is an example of a person who lost some of his long-term memory. In addition, this client has severe short-term memory deficits and is not able to recall information over five minutes.

There is also a distinction between verbal and visual-spatial memory. Verbal memory refers to information that is either read or heard. Reading information in this text (assuming you are wide-awake and concentrating) is employing your verbal short-term memory ability. Remembering the figures in this book may be a combination of both verbal and spatial memory because some of the information is written and other parts pictorial. Spatial memory also refers to recalling information that is seen in a three-dimensional space. When cabinetmakers look at a kitchen for remodeling purposes, they are imagining certain cabinets fitting into a certain space. The space involves three dimensions: height, width, and depth. If this person eyeballs a microwave oven fitting into a certain space, he or she is employing spatial memory by recalling the size of a space and matching it with the visualization of the microwave oven. Verbal and spatial memory are not independent functions but work as a part of a system involving sensory input, attentional skills, problem-solving, and memory ability. Other useful distinctions can involve memory with a context (e.g., an informational paragraph) and random items (e.g., a list of unassociated words). Depending upon a job goal, different effects of memory concerns can have significant vocational implications.

Vocational implications

1. It is important to assess the job tasks and settings for the types of memory skills that are required. Depending upon the client's particular deficits, compensatory means may need to be developed for a particular task or set of tasks.
2. Knowing the client's memory strengths and weaknesses can assist with the appropriate training approach. A person, who may have good visual and spatial memory but significant verbal memory problems, may benefit from being shown tasks rather than being told how to execute a task.
3. Taking a compensatory approach to memory remediation may be helpful. A data entry job, for example, may require the client to repeat a sequence of steps. If a client has verbal memory deficits, the sequence of steps may be jumbled, with some steps missing. The client may benefit from a list of steps that can be immediately reviewed and

circumvent the problem of jumbling or missing steps in the sequence. Some clients with better visual-spatial memory profit from a pictorial sequences of steps to be taken (e.g., on an assembly job) above their workbench or desk.

4. Exercising the memory by use of general word drills or computer cognitive retraining tasks is not likely to generalize to the work setting. Developing compensatory means that are relevant to particular tasks can be most efficient (e.g., taping instructions, having the next day's tasks faxed to a client's home the night before for review, or using categorical cues for remembering items).

5. In many rehabilitation settings, the client is trained in the use of a memory book. Working with the employer or co-workers on using this memory book at the site can make the client more functional. This memory book, in essence, becomes the client's prosthetic memory. Use of the book becomes more habitual if the client is repeatedly trained on use of the book and its contents. Other memory aids are reviewed in the Assistive Technology chapter of this text.

Visual-perceptual abilities

The concept

Related to spatial memory skills is the area of visual-spatial and perceptual-motor integration skills. These visual-spatial abilities relate to the capacity to analyze spatial relationships and make sense of depth and space parameters. Perceptual-motor integration skills refer to the ability to perceive stimuli, formulate a representation of those visual stimuli, remember them, and translate those stimuli into a motor response (e.g., drawing a picture of an object that is presented visually). Visual disturbances can occur after brain injury. The famous case of the person with visual agnosia in (Oliver Sack's well-read book of clinical vignettes entitled *The Man Who Mistook His Wife For a Hat*)[16] describes a distinct case of a person whose vision was intact but whose visual processing abilities were damaged. As mentioned earlier, these visual processing skills are located primarily in the occipital lobes. Being able to see objects and make sense of them requires a combination of both intact vision and cortex to interpret the input. Depth perception, size estimation, and coordinating the hands and feet with visual input are all part of this particular area of cognitive functioning.

Vocational implications

1. Visual skills are necessary in trades such as carpentry, graphic design, mechanics, machine operation, quality control, product inspection, etc. Analysis of job requirements that call for strong visual capabilities

(e.g., an airline pilot) along with other skills may make it more complicated to develop an appropriate rehabilitation approach.

2. Vision and the visual pathways should always be assessed in clients with traumatic brain injury. Medical procedures are available to correct some problems such as double vision. An eye examination may assist you in finding out whether a new pair of glasses or contacts will solve the problems related to visual abilities or you are observing more central nervous system problems in visual processing.

3. The work environment can also be modified to assist with visual difficulties. Something as simple as increasing the available light or organizing the client's work desk or station can make visual processing easier. Day- vs. night-shift positions may need to be considered.

4. Accuracy checks of a person's work may help not only in the visual area but also in all the other areas mentioned. Attention to visual details can be impaired in clients with brain injury and feedback from a supervisor or co-worker can assist the client in proofing his work and increasing his productivity.

Language and communication skills

The concept

The majority of brain injury rehabilitation programs have speech and language pathologists on staff to evaluate and treat clients with language and communication deficits. The neuropsychological evaluation does not always yield a wealth of data in the language and communication area. You may need to ask the neuropsychologist for specific information and/or obtain more specific assessment from a speech pathologist. Language comprehension and language output are two areas that are often assessed in a neuropsychological evaluation. Problems in these areas are often referred to as aphasia. A person may be able to understand things that people say or things that are written, but have difficulty verbalizing or writing his thoughts. This is an expressive aphasia. A receptive aphasia refers to problems understanding information that is written or spoken. Sometimes clients with a TBI are able to understand well, but have problems articulating the words themselves. This is a motor-speech impairment. Speech and language skills are intact, but the motor ability to initiate talking is impaired. Certain common difficulties experienced in the language area are less obvious — clients can be challenged by complex or run-on sentences.

There are other communication problems that occur after brain injury. Speech and language pathologists label these difficulties as problems with *pragmatics*. As mentioned earlier in the behavioral disinhibition section, pragmatics refers to conversational problems in effectively communicating (e.g., use of gestures, conversational turn taking, or organization of conversation's content).

Vocational implications

1. A person with brain injury who has lost many verbal output skills may need to be placed in an area that tends to be more nonverbal. A schoolteacher may no longer be able to conduct a class lecture in history, but may perform well doing the tasks of a librarian or as a one-to-one tutor for a student. A person who may have a problem with the pragmatics of conversation may do better working alone rather than with a number of co-workers or customers.
2. Certain language deficits after brain injury can be subtle. To the casual observer, these problems may not be visible. In planning for employment or re-employment, it would be important for employers to know the nature of any language problems so that mislabeling does not unnecessarily occur on the job site.
3. In vocational counseling sessions or job-site communication, clients with language concerns might be asked to paraphrase the essence of a discussion or communication to be sure they received it accurately.

Complex problem-solving and adaptive reasoning: executive functioning

The concept

As mentioned earlier, the highest forms of cognitive processing are those of complex problem-solving and abstract reasoning. The frontal lobes are often associated with these functions but these abilities are more likely a combined function of many areas of the brain and many types of skills. Stuss and Benson[17] state that processing at this level involves anticipation of events, goal selection, pre-planning, and self-monitoring. Many clients with brain injury lose the ability to self-correct their behavior and errors due to a shallow sense of self-awareness. They may unknowingly repeat their errors. Problems with this higher-order processing can result in an impaired new learning ability and inability to benefit from feedback and deduce a solution from provided details. Organizing activity in a logical sequence and being efficient with job tasks are included in this cognitive processing function. Higher-order functions require organizing an activity, initiating it, and modifying direction with incoming feedback. After brain injury, learning capacity can become more limited due to issues in this area. Training, job site modifications, or adaptive equipment may be required to compensate for these deficits.

General cognitive flexibility and efficiency

The concept

Similar to complex problem-solving is the ability to think flexibly and to do so efficiently. When faced with problems of everyday life, most of us are able to come up with one or two solutions to a problem. To create alternative solutions, one must be able to abandon one method in favor of another. Individuals after brain injury may lose this capacity to change their problem-solving strategy. Perseveration is a term that is sometimes used to describe a person who employs the same incorrect strategy to a problem and does not benefit from feedback. The ability to cognitively process multiple inputs (e.g., listening to verbal instructions while executing a task, coordinating eye-hand movements, and blocking out distracting stimuli) may be considered another example of the ability to process information flexibly and quickly. An aspect of cognitive flexibility is this capacity to process diverse information expediently.

Vocational implications

1. Work trials, job stations, or on-the-job training situations are very important to examine new learning capacity in the client with brain injury. They will also help in assessing the person's ability to adjust efficiently to novel situations and perform multiple tasks simultaneously. It is important to carefully observe where problem-solving deficits impede job performance. These are often difficult to assess and sometimes even more difficult to remediate.
2. The more familiar the task the better. Relying on overly learned tasks minimizes the need for new learning. If there are new tasks to be trained, much repetition and modeling may be needed.
3. Training a client with brain injury in a method of problem-solving that is job or task specific is helpful. Individuals with a TBI may have difficulty transferring learned skills from one group of tasks or job setting to another.
4. Clients who have problem-solving deficits will likely need supervision by co-workers or other supervisors. Job coaches or co-worker trainers can be helpful by providing feedback and cues to keep the client from making too many errors. The co-worker as trainer strategy reviewed in Chapter six has a number of tools to assist individuals in positions requiring higher-order executive functioning and cognitive flexibility.

Limitations of neuropsychological assessment in vocational planning

Many of us would sometimes prefer having a crystal ball or some other way of minimizing the amount of work that is required when it comes to lengthy and complex vocational rehabilitation. In planning for work access for clients with traumatic brain injury, tools that help separate the wheat from the chaff relative to vocational rehabilitation steps are appreciated. Neuropsychological evaluations can be of assistance in making better decisions about jobs and job tasks that are appropriate for the client. Certainly if neuropsychological assessment worked like a crystal ball, the current chapter would be unnecessary. Neuropsychological assessment has predictive limitations relative to a person's ability for everyday tasks and work behaviors. The evaluation, therefore, should be considered a compass that points one in an approximate direction toward the goal of obtaining the best fit between job tasks and a client's cognitive assets and deficits.

Relevance to everyday functioning

Implied in the practice of neuropsychological assessment is the assumption that test results have something to do with what the person does on a daily basis. Each result is just a sample of behaviors from which one generalizes to what a person can be expected to do in the real world. Ultimately, for example, one would like to see a client's performance on the Wechsler Memory Scale be highly predictive of this client's ability to remember a set of instructions given by a construction foreman. It would also be helpful to know if the Trail Making Test could predict to what extent a truck driver might be able to return to time-pressured, long-haul jobs. We would also all be quite happy to know if the Category Test could tell if a trial lawyer could effectively present a case. We live, unfortunately, in a very complex world with a seemingly infinite amount of variables to account for daily performance. In this regard, neuropsychological assessment falls short of being able to make such direct predictions. As mentioned before, the neuropsychological evaluation should be looked upon as a compass rather than a map of a person's daily behavior.

Two problems exist in the prediction of everyday behaviors from neuropsychological performance tests. One may overestimate the impact of neuropsychological deficits on everyday experience. Some individuals perform poorly on tests yet are able to carry out a number of everyday tasks (e.g., driving without getting lost, performing complex sequences of behavior, or carrying out job tasks) which would not be expected based upon the testing results. This may be due to a number of factors. A person may have a lot of experience with a particular task and, therefore, this task becomes overlearned and routine. There may be cues in the environment that assist the client with a particular task (e.g., a friendly co-worker who reminds the client about doing the particular part of a task). There may have been factors that influenced the testing session itself, such as fatigue, pain difficulties, or distractibility. Usually, the person who administers the test evaluates these factors fairly. Alternatively, based upon the neuropsychological results, one can underestimate the deficits that a person will have in everyday functioning. Bear in mind that the testing situation is structured, performed in a quiet and distraction-free environment, and tests maximal performance. Real-world situations are infrequently quiet, structured, and friendly to the person to encourage best performance. Therefore, you may find a client becoming quite overwhelmed and performing poorly in real-life challenges, even though the test results looked acceptable.

Recommendations

The ultimate goal of a neuropsychological assessment is to be able to make accurate predictions of a client's ability to carry out everyday behaviors and job tasks. Assessment findings, therefore, should not be the only source or the primary source of information to make such predictions. For example, although it is important for the health care professional to be aware of a client's ability to plan, organize, and efficiently execute tasks to make decisions about independent living, other sources of information need to be taken into account. *In vivo* community assessment with observational data can be useful to augment neuropsychological information. You may wish to set up a job try-out or trial (see Chapter six for fuller discussion) to observe a client's ability to carry out certain job tasks. You may be able to build upon this situation by adding complexity to the tasks, as well as cues and other prompts to help. Situational assessment, therefore, can be the cornerstone upon which a good vocational plan can be built. This is particularly important when the neuropsychological findings are questionable.

In examining a work trial it is important to take a fairly close look at the client's abilities. A person can fail on a particular job for many reasons. It is important to discover at what point a client has difficulties. The neuropsychological evaluation can emphasize high-risk areas (e.g., a client may have problems handling multiple input). It will likely be the task of the rehabilitationist to translate these concerns into hypotheses about what may occur on the job (e.g., the client may have difficulties as a receptionist because of customers arriving and telephone calls occurring simultaneously). It is important to work with the neuropsychologist to translate test findings into probable or possible real-world concerns.

Utilizing a neuropsychologist in vocational planning

Who is qualified to conduct a neuropsychological evaluation?

A wide spectrum of practitioners offer neuropsychological services. The range includes people who have taken a course in neuropsychological assessment or have attended a three-day workshop on some aspect of neuropsychology to individuals who obtained the diplomate from the American Board of Professional Psychology/American Board of Clinical Neuropsychology (ABPP/ABCN). Non-neuropsychologists are not expected to know the fine differences between the training backgrounds of different kinds of psychologists. Therefore, it is recommended that when making a referral to a neuropsychologist, the person referring should investigate and research which professional will be most appropriate.[18]

There are some basic requirements that one may wish to consider in choosing a neuropsychologist to evaluate a client who you may be seeking to return to work. They are:

1. The qualified neuropsychologist should have a foundation in test construction and psychometric theory. Most neuropsychological tests have certain properties that make them good vs. non-useful. These properties include various forms of reliability and validity. To understand these concepts, the neuropsychologist should be grounded in the empirical construction of tests. Most manuals for psychological tests contain this type of information. At the very least, the neuropsychologist should understand and be able to evaluate the information that appears in these test manuals.

2. The qualified neuropsychologist should have experience in the standardized administration, scoring, and interpretation of tests. There is some variation as to who administers and scores the different kinds of neuropsychological tests. In some cases, a trained psychometrist administers and scores the tests, while the neuropsychologist interprets the tests and writes the report. Nevertheless, it is important for the neuropsychologist to have a strong background in the standard administration and scoring of tests. This often occurs in the psychologist's graduate training program. The neuropsychologist should know how a particular test is used, in which context a test is most appropriate to utilize, and the extent to which a test will apply to a particular client.

3. The qualified neuropsychologist should have experience in applying neuropsychological tests to populations with neuropsychological impairments. Interpreting test results within the population with TBI can be confusing since there often is no distinct pattern of test results. It is often helpful, therefore, to have had experience interpreting results from different types of brain injury. Knowing the text profile for clients with a stroke or particular type of tumor can help the neuropsychologist in discriminating a profile of scores from a client with traumatic brain injury.

4. The qualified neuropsychologist should have experience in writing comprehensive reports based upon a full set of neuropsychological test results. Many psychologists get limited academic training in how to write a report, or how to write clearly and concisely. It seems that much emphasis in graduate education is on content rather than style. Further training in report writing often comes as a matter of experience and post-graduate supervision. Translating test results into a cohesive report is a combined art and science. Therefore, to answer clinical questions, a neuropsychologist who has test result translation abilities may be desirable.

Training background of a neuropsychologist

As mentioned earlier, the training and background of those who call themselves clinical neuropsychologists can be broad. Many clinical neuropsychologists are licensed clinical psychologists with specialty training and experience in neuropsychology. Graduate training in clinical psychology usually covers a broad range of diagnostic and psychological intervention training. Some choose to specialize in neuropsychology. Many of those who fit this category have had coursework in clinical neuropsychology, clinical neuroanatomy and neurophysiology, test construction, and psychometric theory. Academic coursework is followed with clinical practicum experiences in the administration, scoring, and interpreting of test results. State licensure requirements and accreditation standards through national organizations like the American Psychological Association often guide the graduate training program curriculum. Most programs that are accredited by the American Psychological Association require at least a one-year, full-time pre-doctoral internship at an APA-approved training site. During this internship training, the psychology intern may also obtain specialty training in neuropsychology. There are also specialty post-doctoral fellowships in clinical neuropsychology that last between one and three years. Finally, there are some new graduate training programs specifically for clinical neuropsychology.

There is also a specialty board certification for neuropsychology. This is administered through the American Board of Professional Psychology (ABPP)/American Board of Clinical Neuropsychology (ABCN). There are a number of individuals across the country that possess ABPP/ABCN credentials. These are people who initially send an application to ABPP. After approval, they send in work samples. Following work sample approval, they submit to an oral examination by other ABPP/ABCN credentialed neuropsychologists. The American Board of Professional Neuropsychology is another national body that offers a board certification in neuropsychology for which the "ABPN" is the terminal designation. This latter board uses a similar credentialing process.

There are a number of training seminars and workshops given throughout the country in the area of clinical neuropsychology. These are primarily meant as tune-ups or ways to bolster one's education in the area of neuropsychology, and generally not meant as criteria-based training for clinical competence in the field. The American Psychological Association[18] recently published a definition of what is required for an individual to be called a neuropsychologist. The essential elements are as follows:

1. successful completion of systematic didactic and experiential training in neuropsychology and neuroscience at a regionally accredited university;
2. two or more years of appropriate supervised training applying neuropsychological services in a clinical setting;

3. licensing and certification to provide psychological services to the public by the laws of the state or province in which he or she practices;
4. review by one's peers as a test of these learned competencies.

Different theoretical orientations in neuropsychology

As you are probably well aware, few fields of study exist that are without some disagreement regarding theory and practice. This is true for the field of clinical neuropsychology. A number of approaches or camps have emerged. Each camp developed out of a specific history or tradition and each has its proponents. There are many ongoing debates that center around which approach is the most preferred or useful and under what conditions.

First, distinctions between *fixed* vs. *flexible* battery methods need to be made. Fixed battery approaches are those that employ a standard set of measures or procedures across clients. This allows for comparison of results to various norms, with and without known neurologic impairment. In the flexible battery approach, a set of measures is chosen for usage in each individual case. It may include some tests that are given uniformly, as well as other measures that suit a particular referral question. It is thought that questions about a case may be answered more specifically in this way.

As noted in Figure 11, the two most common batteries are the Halstead-Reitan Neuropsychological Test Battery and the Luria-Nebraska Neuropsychological Test Battery. The two names associated with the batteries (Fixed Batteries Are From Mars, Flexible Batteries Are From Venus) are Ralph Reitan and Charles Golden, respectively. Often these two batteries are augmented by other cognitive tests such as the Wechsler Adult Intelligence Scale (WAIS-R, WAIS-III). The two most well-known approaches in the flexible battery camp are the **hypothesis testing approach** that has been championed by Muriel Lezak, Ph.D., and the **Boston process approach** whose main spokesperson is Edith Kaplan, Ph. D.

The bottom line is that in the hands of a skilled clinical neuropsychologist, whose training in rehabilitation and knowledge of traumatic brain injury are strong, one is likely to have clinical questions answered appropriately. All four approaches could equally be ineffective or inappropriate in the hands of an inexperienced clinician. Obtaining information about the approach of the neuropsychologist you plan to use will be very important when determining if this is the professional who will be the best resource.

Poorly qualified specialists

Please refer to the previous section on the training and background of the neuropsychologist and note that if these qualifications are absent, you may question whether or not it is appropriate to obtain that individual's services. It should also be noted that psychologists are bound by ethical standards and principles. Misrepresenting one's expertise would be an ethical and professional violation. Therefore, there are few psychologists who would

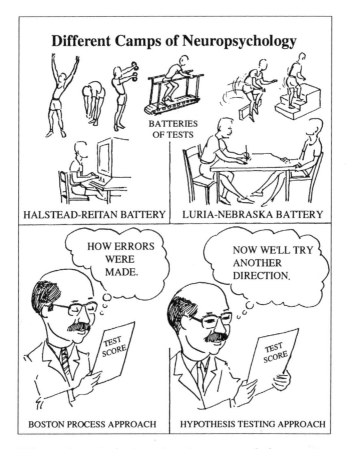

Figure 11 Different theoretical orientations in neuropsychology.

call themselves clinical neuropsychologists if they did not have the appropriate training or background to do so.

Most important is whether or not the psychologist who is involved in an assessment can competently provide input and recommendations that are needed for vocational planning purposes. Many can report test scores, but interpreting scores requires greater skill and expertise. For example, a person who only attends a three-day workshop on a particular neuropsychological test battery usually does not have adequate training to translate test scores into meaningful data for vocational purposes.

Some psychologists and other professionals (e.g., psychiatrists, neurologists, other rehabilitation professionals) may not have a firm foundation in test construction and psychometrics. It is vitally important to understand the characteristics of a test and to appropriately interpret the score based on these characteristics. Infrequently, a practitioner may rig-up a test for a particular client to answer a specific question. The problem with this approach is that no reference group exists for comparing performance on such a homespun task. There are hundreds of tests available to the psychologist, and the field runs the risk of continually reinventing the neuropsychology test wheel. The competent neuropsychologist will choose tests that are constructed with strong methodological rigor.

There are also neuropsychologists who do an excellent job in diagnosing a problem, but may be weak in the area of translating such results into statements that are meaningful to the vocational counselor. Experience and background in rehabilitation can bridge this gap between test results and the client's clinical picture. Combining statistical information with clinical experience is one helpful method of translating neuropsychological test results into statements that are relevant for vocational planning.

Selection recommendations

It may be important for you to identify a neuropsychologist for your client during the process of vocational counseling and planning. You might compare this to shopping for a new or used car. The following ideas may be helpful:

1. Formulate your questions clearly. It is important to know beforehand exactly what you want from a neuropsychological assessment (i.e., do not walk into a "car deal" without knowing exactly what you want).
2. Inquire through your colleagues. You probably are not the first person to try to identify a good neuropsychologist. Many of your colleagues and co-workers can be of great help in directing you toward the right person or keeping you away from neuropsychologists who do not have the training and experience you desire.
3. Contact local rehabilitation hospitals. If a hospital does not have a rehabilitation medicine unit, check with one that does. They usually will be aware of a neuropsychologist at their hospital or one that consults for the hospital who can provide a rehabilitation-oriented neuropsychological evaluation. A neuropsychologist who has functioned as a member of a brain injury treatment team is particularly helpful.
4. Inquire through your state psychological association about recommended individuals. Most state psychological associations maintain a list of psychologists, by region, who work with certain populations and have specific kinds of expertise.
5. Inquire through national associations that deal with neuropsychology. The International Neuropsychological Society (INS), the National Academy of Neuropsychologists (NAN), Division 40 (Clinical Neuropsychology) of the American Psychological Association (APA), and the American Congress of Physical Medicine and Rehabilitation (ACRM) can be good resources for locating a neuropsychologist in your area. These are national organizations that maintain membership lists and usually have the lists broken down by subspecialties.

6. Inquire through your local or state brain injury association or the National Brain Injury Association. You can usually talk with an individual who can help you identify neuropsychologists in your local area. They may also provide recommendations based upon consumer input as to an appropriate individual to conduct an assessment.
7. Request a vita or resume. Just as you would obtain literature on a car that you wish to buy, you may want to look at the qualifications of a neuropsychologist before you employ his or her services. From that individual's vita, you may be able to interview the prospective neuropsychologist about certain training and background areas that you deem important for your client's sake. You may also wish to ask how many cases or what types of cases the identified neuropsychologist handled that are relevant to the problem you are presenting.
8. Give the chosen neuropsychologist technical input if this person is weak in an area of concern. If you have a client with a certain type of disability or neurologic disorder, you may be aware of articles that may help familiarize the neuropsychologist with the problem. Doing research on your client's condition may not be at the top of your list of things to do; however, maintaining relevant and important articles may become useful in the future.

Questions to ask a neuropsychologist: suggested approaches

What the neuropsychologist needs

1. Provide the neuropsychologist with a letter that lists questions you would like answered by the neuropsychological evaluation. It is generally helpful for the neuropsychologist to know ahead of time what questions should be addressed in the evaluation. This may alter the type of tests that are administered, particularly for those who do not use a fixed-battery approach. It is important to be as concrete as possible with your questions. The report you receive and/or a cover letter will, consequently, contain the specific answers to your questions. Should you need to further discuss the evaluation, you will then have a report that will assist you in formulating more questions.
2. Providing a job description with a listing of tasks involved in the job, as well as within the work environment, is helpful. Translating test results to actual work behaviors is difficult; therefore, if you know ahead of time the job or jobs with their assigned critical tasks (and the possibility of assistance with some tasks) that you may be targeting, it can be quite helpful to the neuropsychologist. Clients after brain injury often have difficulties due to a work environment in which there may be considerable people traffic, distractions, noise, or other

variables that can alter job performance. A client's cognitive skills may, therefore, be tenuous in such an environment and the neuropsychologist may wish to offer some recommendations in this area. A complete job analysis according to U.S. Department of Labor criteria can be even more helpful—job descriptive information on more than 12,000 jobs is available through the Directory of Occupational Titles (U.S. Department of Labor, 1991), but is becoming less current.

3. Ask the neuropsychologist for what types of records he or she desires. When you are sending a client to be evaluated, the neuropsychologist often requires a set of medical records or other previous evaluations to obtain background information that may be relevant to the test results. Not all neuropsychologists are the same with regard to the information they need. Therefore, it is important to ask before the evaluation what records should be provided.

4. Request a time frame within which you would like to have the evaluation completed and the vocational plan developed. Most individuals tend to work more efficiently with clear deadlines and you probably do not wish to be waiting for a report to make a decision. Therefore, it is sometimes helpful to clarify these logistics. A good neuropsychological report does take time, particularly if you are asking many specific questions. Some neuropsychologists use a brief rating sheet for identifying cognitive areas of strength and concern until the complete report can be prepared.

What is helpful to the vocational rehabilitation professional?

1. Ask the neuropsychologist what client assets can be capitalized upon. Many reports, not only by neuropsychologists but also by physicians and other health care professionals, tend to be oriented exclusively toward a client's deficits. This is only part of the story. Inquiring about the client's assets can often be more helpful than dwelling on what the client is unable to do, particularly when planning for work access. Traumatic brain injury does not always affect all areas of cognition and there are usually areas that are relatively preserved or represent old learning. These are areas that can be emphasized in trying to find a match between a job and the client's abilities.

2. Ask which areas of deficit are amenable to remediation and to what extent recovery/training can contribute to change. The neuropsychologist may be able to state functions that are expected to improve due to spontaneous recovery or can be assisted by compensatory strategies or other means. This is important to know if you find a job that requires a task in which the client has some deficits, but for which a reasonable degree of improvement can be expected. Depending upon a client's time since injury, different degrees of spontaneous recovery can be expected.

3. Ask what areas of deficit are less likely to change and should be worked around in vocational planning. Some areas of cognitive functioning may be stable and will remain in the impaired range. These are important to know, specifically, since you may be able to plan around such problems. For example, if a client continues to have fine-motor dexterity problems, finding a job that minimizes this kind of work would generally be important to investigate. Often in a case of a traumatic brain injury, there may be several areas of deficit that complicate the process of work access.

4. Ask in what ways particular deficits will impact a particular job's performance. An individual may have a set of cognitive problems that have a minimal effect on performance of job tasks. For example, a person may have some verbal memory deficits but maintains good visual memory abilities, has retained old learning, and possesses adequate motor abilities. Such a person may be able to return to a manual labor type of work and the verbal memory deficit may not greatly impact performance. The same pattern of neuropsychological deficits in a person who is attempting to return to secretarial work may, however, present a major barrier to re-employment. Again, it will be important for you to clarify and discuss with the neuropsychologist particular situations to help the neuropsychologist make predictions about future job performance.

5. Ask what the best strategy may be to train a client for a job task. Depending upon the level of impairment, the neuropsychologist may provide you with some leads as to the best ways to train a client. Some may need verbal and written cues, while others may benefit more from visual presentations of instructions. Others may need instructions given in smaller chunks, augmented with a memory system, to recall steps in the task. These kinds of strategies may be developed in discussions with the neuropsychologist.

6. Ask how the client will handle a situation with multiple inputs. A cardinal feature of traumatic brain injury is that the client is unable to think well under conditions in which more than one thing is happening. You may be able to train a client on a particular job task, but not anticipate other stimuli or distractions in the immediate environment. Therefore, it will be important to know the degree to which a client is able to handle these concerns. This may come from direct observations of the client in the job situation; however, the neuropsychologist may be able to offer some general guidelines regarding the functions with which a client is likely to be more successful.

7. Ask what modifications could be made to the client's work environment to enhance productivity/longevity on the job. Through discussions with the neuropsychologist, you may be able to brainstorm ideas together about changes in the work environment that may enhance performance.

8. If a job coach or co-worker trainer is available, ask how such a person can best be used in directly training or mentoring the client. The neuropsychologist may be able to tell you specific tasks in which the client is likely to need one-to-one assistance. These deficit areas are based upon cognitive impairments that are unlikely to spontaneously recover or for which it may be difficult for the client to compensate independently. If there are behavioral difficulties, such as excessive verbalizations, the trainer may need to cue the client about this problem or employ other strategies. This is information that may be gathered by the neuropsychologist, but also through your own observations and those of significant others.

9. Ask if there are any behavioral problems that may interfere with job performance. Throughout the neuropsychological evaluation, many observations of the client are made that may be relevant to a particular job task. The way in which a client approaches a neuropsychological test reflects how he might approach a particular job task. Impulsivity, impatience, low frustration tolerance, problems with sustained attention, temper problems, and other traits may certainly be behaviors of concern at a job site.

10. Ask if there are any substance abuse issues that may interfere with job performance. You may have already ascertained this information; however, it is fairly standard for a neuropsychologist to obtain this type of background data for use in evaluating the test results. The neuropsychologist or psychologist may be able to give you recommendations about treatment options for substance-abusing clients. Vocational planning may be contingent upon your client enrolling in drug or alcohol treatment.

11. Ask if there are any established family/marital issues that may interfere with job performance. Psychosocial issues are central to a person's ability to function at work. Although some persons can distinctly separate work from home life, it may be more difficult for the client with a brain injury. Ongoing home conflicts may spill over into the work setting and put the client at risk for losing a job. Referrals to appropriate counseling resources can be made by neuropsychologists familiar with local mental health or rehabilitation system professionals.

12. Ask if there are any social issues that may interfere with job performance. As the neuropsychologist explores a client's social network, an individual's friendships and social/recreational pursuits may become issues to successful work access. If a person's social life extends into the wee hours of the morning, it is unlikely that this client will be alert and highly productive the next day, especially if the client has experienced a brain injury. Social and recreational information is often obtained within the context of a neuropsychological evaluation.

Clients avoiding substance abuse may need consultation about new social directions.

13. Ask to what extent physical fatigue and/or pain difficulties will impact job performance. Fatigue difficulties are a common feature of traumatic brain injury. They do not seem to be easily treated, or necessarily improve over time. The neuropsychological evaluation usually occurs over the course of 6 to 8 hours and can be a test of both performance and fatigability. Pain behaviors can also be readily observed over the course of a full day's testing. Such pain difficulties may interfere with test performance and give some indication of how these problems will impact job performance. These observations may be helpful to you in further vocational planning and rehabilitation efforts.

14. Ask for recommendations the neuropsychologist can make on a particular case. In your cover letter to the neuropsychologist, it may be helpful to include what you think may be potential recommendations and ask the neuropsychologist to respond. You may wish to direct the neuropsychologist's recommendations to particular vocational, psychosocial, or other areas relevant to your vocational planning. Ask for specifics when possible. You may need to follow-up on recommendations by clarifying them with the neuropsychologist.

In closing, treat the neuropsychologist's findings as hypotheses and not facts. The neuropsychological evaluation does not provide all the answers that one may wish to have about a particular client. Testing is only a sample of the client's behavior and offers leads as to what may occur in an actual job situation. Combining the neuropsychologist's test results with information you have already gathered or later observe can be an excellent combination for providing better vocational planning and services. Neuropsychological testing, by itself, as discussed may over- or underestimate aspects of real-life functioning.

Examples of neuropsychological reports

The following examples represent two types of neuropsychological reports. The first one is quite detailed, but would require a great deal of clarification for the vocational counselor to use it in vocational planning. The second report was generated as a result of a referral from a vocational rehabilitation counselor who did a good job of asking specific questions. These examples are not intended to suggest one report is necessarily better than the other. Rather, these examples are meant to underscore the need for making reports specific to a context. Again, the vocational rehabilitation counselor's responsibility is to contribute to the final neuropsychological report by posing specific questions and making clear report expectations.

A sample report that requires clarification

The following is an example of a neuropsychological evaluation that was conducted on a 34-year-old client who sustained a traumatic brain injury. This report was chosen since the assessment was requested by a vocational rehabilitation counselor to assist in planning for reemployment.

Some features of this report are worth noting. First, it is rather lengthy. Most of us would not normally sit down for a long period of time to read considerable details that require much translation and clarification. In fact, many of us may jump to the bottom line and look at the summary section only. Although this is not a good practice, in longer reports it is easy to do. The background information section of this report provides some good historical information and is perhaps the report's strength. A symptom review also appears. Second, the report is divided into various subsections on cognitive and emotional functioning. Technical information appears here that is likely more relevant to the neuropsychologist than the vocational rehabilitation counselor. Third, the summary and conclusion section do not directly address many vocational issues that may be of interest to a counselor who is attempting to find an appropriate job placement for a client. Cognitive re-training is recommended; however, this term has so many meanings that it is difficult to know what the neuropsychologist means. No specific recommendations are made. In this case, the vocational counselor will need to contact the neuropsychologist and use considerable conferencing to understand the results and their implications for vocational rehabilitation.

REPORT OF NEUROPSYCHOLOGICAL EVALUATION
(Note: Names and background have been altered to maintain anonymity of the client and neuropsychologist)

Birth Date:	1-12-63
Evaluation Dates:	2-20 and 2-27-97
Age:	34 years
Name:	Shelley Smith
Psychometrist:	Nancy Jones, B.A.
Neuropsychologist:	Phillip Johnson, Ph.D.

Background information

Shelley Smith is a 34-year-old, right-handed female referred for neuropsychological testing by her vocational counselor, James Wong. The purpose of this evaluation is to determine Ms. Smith's strengths and weaknesses, personality orientation, and emotional stability to identify appropriate vocational goals to develop an appropriate program leading to those goals.

The client was in her usual state of good health when on 8-13-93 she was involved in a motor vehicle accident, whereupon she was taken to Community General Hospital trauma center. She arrived in a coma. After initial care at the Intensive Care Unit, she was discharged to the Eastside Medical Center for continued therapies. During this hospitalization, the client gained abilities to stand, walk, run, and take care of her own activities of daily living. She was discharged to the local care of a neurologist, Peter Larson, M.D. and her physiatrist, George Banks, M.D.

At the time of her discharge, Ms. Smith continued to have profound deficits of short-term memory and some behavioral disturbances. Her EEG was grossly abnormal and she was maintained on Dilantin. She had an episode of toxicity on this seizure medication resulting in an episode of blacking out. The patient's family felt it necessary to move her from her own condominium to her parents' home in Seattle. The client was noted to have continued problems with hyperirritability and emotional lability. Nevertheless, medical records indicate that she was progressing in her recovery. She was also noted to have problems taking care of her daily living needs and was unable to return to work.

Ms. Smith was involuntarily re-admitted to Community General Hospital for approximately two weeks in 1995 due to poor impulse control and low frustration tolerance. She could not care for herself or her children on the day of admission and apparently became uncontrollable when her children were removed from her custody and given to her mother. During her hospital stay, neuropsychological testing was obtained at which time her intelligence was considered to be in the dull normal range. On the Halstead-Reitan Neuropsychological Battery, the client was impaired on 70% of the tests administered. She showed problems with abstract thinking and problem-solving as well as memory, learning, and behavioral controls. The evaluation revealed moderate to severe loss of intellectual and adaptive abilities. It was recommended that she be enrolled in a cognitive re-training program.

Social background is as follows: Ms. Smith is the fourth of nine siblings. She was described as having been active, healthy, and rapid in her development. Medical records indicate that from childhood her home life was deprived and chaotic. She was frequently without adequate nutrition according to some reports. Her father was killed in a shooting incident when the client was 13 years old. As a result of his death, she was referred for psychiatric evaluation but refused to talk about her feelings. In 1976, at age 13, the client underwent another psychiatric evaluation. Later that year she was suspended twice from school due to behavior problems. Two years later she had a neck injury related to activity in a physical education class. Medically, the client has a history of a head injury in school in which she knocked herself out and lost sight for three months thereafter. This examiner can find no medical records to substantiate that report from the client. Medical records also show that the client had been found to be within the average range in intellectual testing while in the 8th grade.

[Report continues for another four pages with further background information.]

The client reports that she has been significantly changed as a result of her brain injury. She describes herself as "totally different." When asked to describe her differences she reports the following:

1. "Things bother me easier."
2. "I can't keep my mind on one thing."
3. "I have no activities in my day."
4. "There is a big gap in my memory."
5. The client feels she is less intelligent than she was before the injury and she has concerns that she has forgotten information. She reports that she had been an average or above average student in algebra and English prior to her injury and is now uncertain of what she learns and remembers.
6. The client is aware of lowered self-esteem. Although she formerly worked her way up from an erratic school performance to academic success, she is currently unable to attend school and is worried about her future. She feels that people treat her with less respect than they did when she was a college student and wants very much to return to college and her previous vocational goals.

Observations and interview

Ms. Smith was seen on two occasions for testing, each time for about three hours. Although she had planned to arrive early, she got lost in the hospital, a common occurrence for people coming to this office for the first time. On the second testing session, she was 30 minutes late. Upon questioning, the client states she frequently has trouble judging the time. Ms. Smith was highly cooperative throughout the evaluation. She was well motivated to do her best and persisted at difficult tasks when given encouragement to do so. She asked for repetitions and clarifications of instructions as necessary, but was variable in her ability to comply with task demands. She was frequently unhappy with her own performance and reported greater difficulty in catching onto things as compared with her pre-injury abilities. At times she had trouble interpreting questions and giving simple answers to simple questions.

Tests administered

The evaluation included both quantitative and qualitative measures. The quantitative procedures included the Wechsler Adult Intelligence Scale-Revised, Stroop Test, Trailmaking Test, Wechsler Memory Scale-Revised, California Verbal Learning Test, Symbol Digit Modalities Test, Booklet Category Test, Wisconsin Card Sorting Test, Controlled Oral Word Association Test, Wide Range Achievement Test-Revised, Minnesota Multiphasic Personality Inventory-2, Millon Clinical Multiaxial Inventory-III, and a questionnaire of cognitive symptoms. Qualitative procedures included the clinical interview, observations during testing sessions, and a set of informal measures. All of the procedures were administered by this examiner during the course of approximately six hours of testing time. These results are judged to be an accurate current assessment of Ms. Smith's higher cognitive functions.

Evaluation results

1. General intelligence
Ms. Smith's Verbal, Performance, and Full Scale I.Q. scores measured within the average range. Her scaled scores on the Verbal section range varied from two-thirds of a standard deviation above the mean (Arithmetic), placing her in the 75th percentile down to one standard deviation below the mean (Information), placing her in the 16th percentile. There is a trend of I.Q. increases in both the Verbal and Performance areas as compared with previous testing obtained in June 1985. The increase was statistically significant (i.e., one standard deviation increase) in the Performance area. The increase in the Verbal area failed to reach a level of statistical significance. The client's scores on the Performance section of the WAIS-R ranged from one-third standard deviation above the mean (Picture Completion, Picture Arrangement), placing her in the 63rd percentile down to two-thirds standard deviations below the mean (Block Design, Object Assembly), placing her in the 25th percentile.

2. Executive
This client is able to initiate a plan of action, but has extreme difficulty carrying it out when faced with one or more alternatives or distractors. She loses the goal or mental set established and will often select an inappropriate alternative. She is unaware of her own strategy shifts. She becomes confused by the failure of her activities to be fruitful but has no idea as to the source of the problem. When redirected, she begins a process again, but experiences the same failure to maintain the set. Perseverations at times interfere with her ability to shift the set appropriately. This finding is consistent with the deficits reported on the Categories Test in June 1985.

3. Attention/concentration
Ms. Smith is able to initiate and sustain a mental focus for simple tasks. She is able to screen out irrelevant stimuli and sustain concentration for short periods of time. She is more subject to distraction as tasks increase in complexity. Thus, although she is able to maintain selective attention, she is impaired in the ability to maintain either alternating or divided attention. It is this inability to maintain alternating and divided attention that interferes with her ability to be punctual and perform two simultaneous tasks or two-step tasks.

4. Memory

Ms. Smith's memory is affected by her difficulty with focused attention and the nature of the task. Her ability to learn a word list, however, over the course of five trials is within normal limits. Furthermore, she is able to store and then retrieve such information later in a manner probably consistent with her premorbid abilities. Nevertheless, when asked to listen to a short story or paragraph of information, she is markedly impaired in both short-term retention and 30-minute recall. Although she recalls the general gist of the information, she has lost many of the details when she tells it immediately after hearing it. Thirty minutes later she is aware that she retells "a whole different story." Again, she remembers the primary themes but is unable to retain the specific details. She retained only 73% of the information she had recalled from the initial telling. She was able to accurately reproduce geometric designs on a short-term memory basis without difficulty. Thirty minutes later she remembered only 58% of the original designs, which was quite impaired. Perspective memory (i.e., her ability to carry out intended actions) is interfered with by her attentional disorder and impaired executive functions.

5. Sensory-motor

Sensory perceptual functions are generally within the average range. Nevertheless, results of recent previous visual testing reveal the need for glasses to correct a problem with visual acuity. Auditory acuity was serviceable for purposes of this evaluation. Gait and ambulation were unremarkable. Ms. Smith was able to plan, sequence, and organize motor movements on the Lurian maneuvers. Previous testing revealed bilateral grip strength to be intact.

6. Language

The client has some trouble in comprehending language. She is careful to ask for repetitions and clarifications when she is unsure of instructions or question forms. Her expressive language is impaired by some deficits in language ideation as well as vocabulary selection. She has difficulty organizing her thoughts into words to express ideas and also experiences dysnomia or specific word-finding difficulties. At times she uses vocabulary characteristic of an individual with a two-year college education. However, on other occasions, she is unable to think of simple words and relies on descriptions that may be only partially accurate.

7. Visual-spatial

Ms. Smith demonstrates a constructional dyspraxia with some elements of a thought spatial disorder. She has difficulty organizing visual or spatial information and using visual cues simultaneously and in both visual analysis and synthesis. Her systems for construction that were apparently available in the past are no longer accessible to her. Although she attempts to work systematically and to monitor for quality control, as tasks become more difficult she loses the general gestalt or concept and is able to recognize errors but not correct them. The finding of constructional dyspraxia is consistent with test results obtained earlier.

8. Academics

Ms. Smith is able to solve story problems but has difficulty with aspects of calculation abilities. She is presently in the 27th percentile in arithmetic functions (standard score = 91) on the Arithmetic section of the Wide Range Achievement Test. Given her reported history of successful completion of algebra and other courses in higher level mathematics, she should have been able to find averages, use decimals, and calculate with mixed numbers having different denominators. On the basis of history, her arithmetic abilities are markedly impaired at the present time although consistent with her current intellectual functioning.

Written language reveals a tendency to spell phonetically. Nevertheless, the quality of her written language suggests previously better abilities than those she currently exhibits.

9. Emotion/personality

The client's performance on the MMPI-2 appeared to be a valid one. Her test-taking attitude revealed a tendency toward social nonconformity, which she readily acknowledges in all of her contacts with professionals. She endorsed a high number of unusual items, which is fairly common among individuals with seizure disorders. The profile she endorsed was consistent with a lack of self-confidence and low self-esteem. Individuals who endorse this profile often experience confusion and disorganization. They have difficulty in thinking and concentrating. They may have suicidal ideation; however, it is exceedingly difficult to predict the probabilities of suicide for individuals with this profile. It is common for persons with this profile to spend a great deal of time daydreaming or fantasizing. Some unrealistic ideas as well as excessive fears are frequently present. Like others who present this profile, suspicion and some distrust of others are present. Individuals with her current psychological testing profiles tend toward being shy, withdrawn, anxious, and resentful. They have a tendency toward erratic or impulsive behavior and may exercise poor judgement. This profile is consistent with a relatively recent onset of disorder and is not at all uncommon among brain-impaired persons. Fourteen percent of subjects with this profile have sustained brain impairment.

Summary and conclusions

Ms. Shirley Smith is a 30-year-old, right-handed female who sustained a devastating brain injury. Prior to that time she had successfully completed two years of college in a pre-law program and was working as a bus driver at the time of her accident. That history is particularly noteworthy because of her strength and independence which enabled her to live on her own as an adolescent, survive the trauma of her father's death when she was 13, and organize herself sufficiently to earn her G.E.D. in late adolescence. Although she had come from a very disrupted home environment, Ms. Smith had been proud of her own accomplishments and was highly goal-directed. Ms. Smith has sustained some enormous losses as a result of her brain injury. She has sustained a generalized reduction in cognitive functions as reflected by lowered I.Q. scores as well as impairments in executive function, alternating and divided attention, memory, learning complex tasks, comprehension of higher level or complex ideational units, organizing her thoughts into words, and ability to manipulate objects effectively. The latter deficit may be referred to as a constructional dyspraxia. She has also sustained some impairment in reading and arithmetic.

Ms. Smith is readily confused by the changes in her cognitive functions and is highly resentful of them. She feels as though all of her efforts at bettering herself have been thwarted and that she is treated with disrespect as a result of her disabilities.

This client's disorder of executive function may be the most debilitating of her deficits at the present time. In her daily activities, her inability to maintain a mental set of goal-directed activities frequently results in people labeling her as irresponsible. This client is unable to maintain goal-directed activities that were within her capacity in the past. At present she would be unable to organize herself sufficiently to earn a G.E.D., register for college, etc. She has difficulty organizing her time to catch a bus at a different time, working at a 10-minute timed task without distraction, or performing other organized activities. She is unable to move from task to task or alternate between two tasks, or deal with the distractions of alternating and divided attention. Her impulsivity and perseverations are very much a product of her generalized cognitive dysfunction.

Recommendations

Ms. Smith appears to be an appropriate candidate for a formal cognitive retraining program. Such a program should provide primary emphasis on attention focusing, problem-solving, and establishing a mental set. She needs to learn restructuring, problem-solving, and be able to maintain specific goals. It will be critical for her to learn strategies for recognizing and evaluating alternative approaches to solving a problem. The cognitive retraining program should recognize the neurological basis of her disabilities rather than treat them as behavioral disorders that have either a long-standing or non-neurogenic basis. It is also essential that the cognitive retraining program establishes and communicates goals and objectives with Ms. Smith that are realistic and agreeable to her. It will be important for such a program to clarify for her the relationship between her brain injury and her current disabilities.

It is recommended that Ms. Smith be served by the Cognitive Retraining Program at the Community Service Hospital. The program is highly structured and is able to provide Ms. Smith with rehabilitation of cognitive processes as well as vocational rehabilitation in the form of job stations. There is an emphasis on psychosocial adjustment as well as orientation and information processing. The program is individualized and has as its goals successful vocational placement within the community. This program is also more accessible geographically, a major consideration for Ms. Smith.

Philip Johnson, Ph.D.
Clinical Neuropsychologist

A sample report with vocational planning implications

The following is a letter requesting an evaluation written by a vocational rehabilitation counselor to a neuropsychologist. You will notice a set of fairly specific questions. These questions help structure the second report that is presented. This second neuropsychological evaluation is accompanied by a cover letter that addresses point-by-point the questions that were listed in the referral letter.

The neuropsychological report is again divided into various functional areas; however, within each section is contained a brief description of vocational implications. This can be of assistance in creating a vocational plan. It may also generate further questions for discussion with the neuropsychologist. A summary of the major findings coupled with specific recommendations also appears in this report.

This report is certainly not a golden standard in report writing; however, it represents a step in the right direction for usefulness in vocational planning. The process of using neuropsychological findings in one's work is certainly a two-way street. It will likely take some discussion with the neuropsychologist and an independent vocational rehabilitation assessment to generate an appropriate work access or return-to-work plan. The neuropsychological evaluation is but one information component in finding a good job match for the client with traumatic brain injury.

March 20, 1998

Leigh Taylor Fender, Ph.D., Program Director
Neurorehabilitation Program
Seattle, Washington

RE: Robert T. Bayer
Claim #: S-7732149B377

Dear Dr. Fender:
I am a Rehabilitation Counselor who has been asked by Goode Vocational Systems, Inc., to coordinate medical and vocational services relating to the industrial injury of November 27, 1997 of Mr. Robert T. Bayer.

I have scheduled for you to conduct a neuropsychological evaluation on Mr. Bayer on Tuesday, April 3rd. Your staff as needed may schedule other appointments related to the assessment. To provide you with some background, I am enclosing my correspondence with Dr. Forge regarding Mr. Bayer. I am also sending you a job analysis of the work that he does and a description of a light duty job. As you can see from the correspondence, Mr. Bayer fell while working. He broke his jaw and three ribs. There is now further concern that he may have a post-concussion syndrome and your evaluation is for the purpose of evaluating this possibility. Should your examination conclude that he does have this problem, would you further evaluate the nature of the claimant's cognitive impairment?

After you have examined Mr. Bayer, please send a report with the following information:

1) Your diagnoses based upon your testing.
2) What diagnoses do you find related to the injury of November 27, 1997?
3) Is any treatment recommended? If so, please specify the kind of treatment(s) and for what length of time.
4) What limitations are evident from your testing that could affect this gentleman while he works (such as reduced stamina and endurance, difficulty handling stress, memory impairment, difficulty staying focused, or any other mental processing functions)?
5) Do any individual and/or family functioning dynamics exist which may interface with neuropsychological deficits to further impair employment?
6) Because Mr. Bayer had an elevated blood alcohol at the time of his work injury, please evaluate whether or not this testing reveals evidence that Mr. Bayer has significant problems related to drinking alcohol.
7) Do you anticipate that the claimant will achieve full recovery? If so, please project a date when maximum medical improvement will occur.
8) Please review the enclosed job analysis. Considering the specific work that Mr. Bayer does, do you anticipate that the claimant will be able to cognitively perform this job, and if so, when?
9) Please review the enclosed light duty job description. Could he return to work doing this job sooner, from a cognitive capacity perspective? If yes, when?

Please address any other issues you feel relevant to this case. Thank you for your time and considerate attention. If you have any questions, please feel free to call me at 555-1234.

Sincerely,

Lynn Graf, M.S., C.R.C.
Rehabilitation Counselor
Goode Vocational Systems, Inc.

REPORT OF NEUROPSYCHOLOGICAL EVALUATION
(Note: The following is an abbreviated version of the report.
Names and background have been altered to maintain
anonymity of the client and neuropsychologist)

Patient Name:	Robert T. Bayer
Claim Number:	S-7732149B377
Date of Birth:	2-7-58
Age at Time of Testing:	40
Date of Evaluation:	4-3-98; 4-4-98
Education:	High School Graduate
Occupation:	Janitorial
Handedness:	Right
Psychometrist:	Douglas Brown, B.A.
Neuropsychologist:	Leigh Taylor Fender, Ph.D.

Identifying information

Mr. Robert T. Bayer is a 40-year-old male who was injured while working at Charlie's Bakery in Seattle. He was referred to the Neurorehabilitation Program for a comprehensive neuropsychological evaluation by his physician, Dr. Margaret Forge, and by Lynn Graf, M.S., C.R.C., rehabilitation counselor for Goode Vocational Systems, Inc. The following report is based upon a diagnostic interview, review of medical records, and neuropsychological testing results.

Background information

The patient was in his usual state of good health until November 27, 1997 when he was struck on the head with a piece of heavy equipment while doing sanitation work at Charlie's Bakery. The patient reports pushing a machine that got caught on the floor, resulting in the upper portion of the machine falling on top of him. It is reported that the object striking him weighed approximately 58 pounds. The patient recalls all events that led up to the accident, and therefore, there was no retrograde amnesia. Loss of consciousness is estimated to be about 10 to 15 minutes in that the patient recalls waking up and seeing the paramedics. He was taken to the Community Medical Center Emergency Room with a laceration over the right occipital area and a fracture of the left mandible. A head CT scan did not apparently show evidence for significant hemorrhage, mass effect or midline shift. Blood alcohol level drawn at the ER showed a significant level of .172. Mr. Bayer was hospitalized for the next four days and was discharged on 12-1-97 to home. The patient reported not being able to speak English during the first day of admission to CMC, and needed to talk with someone who spoke Italian. The next morning, he recalls being able to again speak English. Initial symptoms at the time of admission included neck, rib, and jaw pain, dizziness, tinnitus, and headaches. He notes having more significant problems with headaches about one week after being discharged from CMC. The headaches were associated with nausea and vomiting.

At the time of the interview for the current evaluation, Mr. Bayer reported symptoms of fatigue, headaches, sleep disturbance, appetite change (largely due to his jaw being wired), increased irritability, depressed mood, crying, difficulty recalling information, misplacing objects, and difficulty carrying through with daily chores. At the time of the interview, the patient had not worked since the injury. The patient reports no previous neurological history, nor previous head trauma. There is no reported history of major physical illness prior to the injury. No seizure history is reported. The patient reports no significant history of drug abuse. He states he will drink twice per week with upwards to having five beers on each occasion. Mr. Bayer noted that when he drinks two to three beers, he now becomes dizzy and sometimes nauseated. The medical records note the patient had a DWI about four years ago. Currently, the patient does not feel he abuses alcohol. He reports no significant psychiatric history prior to the injury.

Mr. Bayer is a high school graduate, with his education being obtained in East Africa. The grade equivalent of his performances was in the B-grade range. The patient states he has had some courses in electrical work and in plumbing. He has worked for Charlie's Bakery for the past four years, and prior to that worked as a store manager in an electrical appliance and materials business for eight years.

The patient has been married for the past 13 years and has two daughters ages 14 and 11, and three sons ages 12, 8, and 6. They live in a rented house. He states he is not yet a U.S. citizen, and has been in the United States for the past five years.

Evaluation procedures

- Halstead-Reitan Neuropsychological Test Battery and Allied Procedures

- Wechsler Adult Intelligence Scale-III
- Consonant Trigrams Test
- Wechsler Memory Scale-III
- California Verbal Learning Test
- Rey Complex Figure Test
- Memory Questionnaire
- Reitan-Indiana Aphasia Screening Test
- Boston Naming Test
- Controlled Oral Word Association Test
- Wisconsin Card Sorting Test
- Minnesota Multiphasic Personality Inventory-2
- Clinical Analysis Questionnaire and the 16PF Inventory

Behavioral observations during test administration

The patient arrived on time for his scheduled testing appointment and was independently ambulatory. There did not appear to be any physical or communication barriers to obtaining a valid test protocol. English is a second language, and therefore, verbal sub-tests may reflect the influence of cultural differences, and consequently will be interpreted conservatively. He appeared alert, understood all tasks, and was cooperative throughout the testing session. Test results are, therefore, a valid representation of his current level of cognitive and psychosocial functioning. On the Head Injury Symptom Checklist, the patient endorsed the following problems: headaches, fatigue, blurred vision, trouble concentrating, bothered by noise, irritability, loss of temper easily, memory difficulty, and anxiety.

Test results

Intellectual functioning

The patient's WAIS-III performance places him in the upper end of the Low Average range of overall intellectual functioning at approximately the 23rd percentile for an age-peer group. This is roughly commensurate with expectation. There did not appear to be evidence of significant decline in general intelligence. Verbal output skills are similar in level to nonverbal skills, and both are in the Low Average to lower end of the Average range (Verbal I.Q. = 92, 30th percentile; Performance I.Q. = 88, 21st percentile). Relatively lower scores were obtained on tests that involve speeded motor tasks, coordination of visual percepts with motoric output, and with verbal abstract reasoning (though the latter ability may be partly due to cultural differences and experience). Strengths appear in the areas of doing mental arithmetic, sequencing events, and logical analysis.

Vocational implications.   It would appear that the patient has previously overlearned and well-rehearsed skills intact. Verbal and nonverbal skills are currently consistent with more manual labor and less verbally oriented tasks. In situations or tasks that require quick motor output in which timed constraints may influence productivity, the patient will likely do more poorly at present. He appears, however, to have a good capacity to learn new, more simple tasks with verbal and nonverbal instruction. Work that requires precision eye-hand coordination should be avoided at present.

Attention/concentration and recent memory functioning

On the WMS-III, the patient obtained a General Memory Index of 108, which is in the upper end of the Average range and suggests no significant global impairment of memory functioning. Specific areas of weaknesses are noteworthy. He maintains better verbal recent memory skill versus visual retention ability. He performs poorly on tasks that involve basic sustained attentional skill. Over a delayed period of time he performs at expectation. Mr. Bayer shows more difficulty on learning verbal information when there lacks a context within which to recall words. He is able to copy and recall complex visual information, though after a delayed period of time, he loses about one-third to one-half of visual details from initial recall. Incidental memory ability (i.e., trying to recall information without prior warning) is impaired. Memory difficulties in everyday situations are significantly high (Memory Questionnaire 77 out of 140; average for those without brain impairment is in the low 20s). He notes frequent problem areas such as forgetting to tell somebody something important, being absent-minded, and losing track of what someone is trying to tell you.

Vocational implications. When giving this individual instructions, it would be helpful to pair verbal cues with visual cues. Both telling the patient instructions and demonstrating the action will benefit his overall performance on the job. It would be important for co-workers and supervisors to repeat information and check with Mr. Bayer to make sure he understands instructions. More repetitive tasks with minimal new learning components should be tried first before moving into more complex instructions that require more memory capacity. Where possible, it would be helpful to have the patient list more complex instructions/tasks. The same type of strategy should also be applied in everyday situations (e.g., generating a grocery list, using an appointment book with a things to do section). It would also be helpful to forewarn this individual of important information to be remembered so that he might expend additional effort to write such information.

Complex problem-solving and adaptive reasoning

On the Category Test the patient performed in the mild range of impairment (72 errors; cutoff is 51 errors), suggesting difficulties in logical analysis and adaptive reasoning ability. This was not a consistent finding in that flexible thinking (Trails B = 60 seconds, no errors; cutoff = 90 seconds) and the ability to apply novel problem-solving strategies (WCST = six out of six categories achieved; 93 correct with 29 errors; 15 = perseverative responses, cutoff = 25 responses) were within normal limits.

Vocational implications. On job tasks that require quick decision making, the patient may perform more poorly and below expectation. The patient should not use heavy machinery in which safety to the worker is a concern at this time, particularly with a combined concern of mild problem-solving difficulty with attentional deficits. With cognitive improvement, it would be important for this individual to have supervision for tasks that require use of heavy machinery similar to those that he operated prior to his injury. This individual is likely able to learn new information and task sequences, so long as there is sufficient repetition of tasks, and the supervision provided to correct errors.

Visuospatial ability and perceptual-motor integration
His ability to organize visual percepts and logically analyze such data is within normal limits. Translating visual percepts into quick motoric responses, as mentioned earlier, is slightly weak. He appropriately interprets visual percepts without error or distortion.

Vocational implications. Should there be a need to retrain this individual into a different occupation, it may be initially beneficial to avoid tasks that require precision and fine-motor output (e.g., electronics parts assembler), or precision eye-hand coordination (e.g., a graphics designer type of position). For his previous position, these findings should not interfere significantly.

Language functioning
There did not appear to be evidence for significant word finding, paraphasias, or motor-speech impairments. Verbal skills for this individual where English is a second language appeared to be good. Fluency of word output appears to be good.

Sensory-motor integrity
One right- and two left-sided tactile suppressions occurred upon bilateral stimulation. One left auditory suppression and four right visual suppressions occurred as well. No consistent pattern of lateralization of deficits was noted. Similarly, on fine tactile stimulation tasks, there were two right- and six left-sided errors. The above appear to suggest further problems with sustaining attention and do not provide strong evidence for central nervous system motor dysfunction.

Vocational implications. See Perceptual-Motor Integration section above.

Psychosocial functioning
The patient's MMPI-2 is technically valid and describes an individual who endorsed several unusual items. This may suggest that the patient currently experiences a significant degree of distress and/or confusion. Six of the 10

clinical scales were elevated beyond the significant cutoff point (scales >T65 in order of elevation were 2, 6, 7, 1, 8, 4). Individuals with similar profiles are described as presenting with a depressed and irritable mood, are anxious, ruminative, worrying, and may have a significant sensitivity to the intentions of others. He may harbor significant anger, frustration, and resentment toward himself and/or others. This may be expressed openly. Significant distress in interpersonal relationships may be reported. On the clinical factors of the CAQ, he had significant elevations on scales that would suggest a high degree of focus upon somatic symptoms, resentment, social withdrawal, and feelings of self-deprecation.

In terms of more enduring interpersonal and psychological characteristics (16PF Inventory), this is a person who may tend to be more generally anxious and tense. This level of anxiety can be aggravated by traumatic events such as the accident he experienced recently. Self-image management is of less importance to this individual. At times in his life, this individual may have had a tendency to test social norms and mores. He may also tend to be more easily annoyed than the general population. He may need less interaction with other individuals, and may prefer to work or be alone, rather than being among larger groups of people. Such profiles are more consistent with those who gravitate toward more mechanical-operative types of jobs, and less similar to those occupations that involve leadership and the ability to influence others.

Vocational implications.   This is an individual who would likely not process information rapidly and efficiently due to difficulties with being preoccupied with thoughts and worries. He would work better in a quieter environment with a minimum of psychological stressors. It would also be important to minimize contact with co-workers with whom the patient historically has had interpersonal conflicts. Depression may be contributing to the psychomotor slowness and attentional difficulties that are present. Previous precautions about working around heavy machinery which present safety issues are again emphasized.

Summary of neuropsychological evaluation

1. Given the absence of retrograde amnesia and loss of consciousness of no more than 15 minutes, the pattern of results would suggest this individual has sustained no more than a mild head injury. He currently presents with post-concussion symptoms that have improved since the time of injury.
2. General intellectual functioning is commensurate with expectation. Visual-motor coordination is weak, whereas sequencing events and information is good.
3. General memory functioning is commensurate with current scores. The most significant finding is that of attentional deficits, which likely

affect other areas of cognitive functioning. Frequent everyday problems of forgetfulness are also reported.

4. Complex problem-solving is mildly impaired.
5. Fine motor coordination and speed are relatively weak at present. Attention difficulties may contribute to these problems as well.
6. Depression, frustration, irritability, and social withdrawal are a significant part of the current clinical picture. He may also have problems with anxious rumination and anger control.

Synthesis

This 40-year-old male likely sustained a mild traumatic brain injury, with post-concussion syndrome in the accident of 11-27-97. He presents with attentional difficulties that affect other higher-order cognitive processing such as complex problem-solving. A clinical depression and focus upon bodily symptoms may also contribute to his current attentional problems. He reports several cognitive problems have improved since the injury. The prognosis for further improvement is good contingent upon treatment of the depression, and re-involvement in pre-injury activities on a gradually increasing basis. In this regard, it is likely this individual could return to his previous responsibilities on the job in time and with further gains.

Recommendations

1. It would be important for the patient to receive aggressive treatment for his depression/anxiety problems. Pharmacological and psychological interventions may be useful in this regard. A trial of antidepressant medication and more behaviorally oriented/directive strategies of treatment are likely to be beneficial.
2. A regimen of physical therapy is highly recommended for this patient. Aerobic conditioning and increasing physical endurance may be helpful for potential disuse/deactivation syndrome and may have the added benefit of assisting with depression, fatigue, and attention difficulties. Physical therapy on a regular basis for three to four weeks, then tapering to a home program, all done within a structured and gradually increasing system may be most beneficial to this patient.
3. A gradual return to work plan should be developed and implemented as soon as possible. It would be important for this patient to begin with no more than .50 time work, then increasing his time to .75, then to full-time over the next six to eight weeks.
4. Given his current cognitive deficits, it would be important for this patient to return to work with more simplified tasks that require more repetition and light duty work. An environment that has fewer distractions than his previous situation would be beneficial. Supervision should be provided that can evaluate his performance and readiness to attempt more difficult tasks.

5. Regular and scheduled appointments with a primary care physician would be important to keep this patient reactivated, and prevent disability due to focus upon physical symptoms.

6. Continued involvement and re-evaluation by vocational experts would be beneficial to also keep the patient active and on track with his re-employment. Should there be initial problems with attention/memory in the job situation, work with a rehabilitation professional (e.g., speech therapist, occupational therapist, rehabilitation psychologist) may be of benefit to provide compensatory strategy training that is specific to the work environment.

Leigh Taylor Fender, Ph.D.
Clinical Neuropsychologist
Neurorehabilitation Program

CC: Margaret Forge, M.D.
       Lynn Graf, M.S., C.R.C.

Cover letter accompanying neuropsychological report

April 15, 1998

Lynn Graf, M.S., C.R.C.
Goode Vocational Systems, Inc.
2001 Odyssey Drive, Suite 2010
Seattle, Washington 98108

RE: Robert T. Bayer
Claim Number: S-7732149B377

Dear Ms. Graf:

Thank you for referring your client, Mr. Robert T. Bayer, to the Neurorehabilitation Program for a neuropsychological evaluation. Enclosed for your review are the neuropsychological findings, vocational implications, clinical impressions, and recommendations for your client based upon my evaluation.

I would like to respond directly to the questions you so well articulated in your letter of March 20, 1998.

1. My diagnoses, based upon review of medical records, diagnostic interview, and neuropsychological testing results, would suggest a mild traumatic brain injury with persisting post-concussion symptoms that are resolving. There also appears to be evidence for a clinical depression present. He did not meet criteria for a major depressive episode (MDE) according to (DSM-IV), but had many features of MDE, and therefore at this

time would qualify for an Adjustment Disorder with depressed mood. I suspect a possible alcohol abuse disorder as well, though the patient's self-report would not substantiate this diagnosis.

2. The head trauma with post-concussion syndrome, and the adjustment disorder with depressed mood are, in my opinion, causally related to the industrial accident of November 27, 1997.

3. Treatment is recommended as stated in my report. This consists of regularly scheduled medical follow-up with Dr. Forge, a trial of antidepressant medication, and possible time-limited behaviorally oriented psychotherapy (eight to 10 sessions). I would also recommend short-term physical therapy (six to eight sessions) for endurance and aerobic training, and then periodic follow-up appointments to monitor a home physical therapy program that would be carried out daily by the patient. I believe if Mr. Bayer has trouble on the job site now or in the future due to attentional or memory difficulties, therapy from a rehabilitation professional (e.g., speech therapy, occupational therapy, rehabilitation psychology) may be in order for a time-limited period that is focused upon specific job task deficits (four to six sessions). Vocational counseling is highly recommended to provide input regarding work return on a gradually increasing basis, and to follow-up post-employment status. This would be done on a weekly, then biweekly basis over the course of the next six to 12 months.

4. Limitations at present include physical fatigue and low endurance, reduced capacity to deal with interpersonal stressors and conflict (e.g., difficulty with irritability and anger control), slowed problem-solving, and attentional difficulties that lead to decreased memory efficiency. These are the primary problems that would limit his full work capacity.

5. I did not see significant familial or psychological deficits outside of those already mentioned that interact significantly with current cognitive limitations. It would, however, be important to monitor any social reinforcement of illness behavior by family members or significant others.

6. In my experience, the combination of alcohol-related injury (i.e., he was found to have an elevated blood alcohol level at the time of his injury), a past record of DWI, the patient's self-report of drinking upward to five beers at a sitting twice per week, and the fact that he notices more impact from alcohol on cognitive functioning after his injury strongly suggests that alcohol abuse problems are significant in this case. I certainly would recommend ongoing alcohol treatment for this patient.

7. Full recovery is difficult to forecast. In terms of his ability to return to his former position as a janitor, in my opinion I believe he could do this contingent upon following the rehabilitation recommendations mentioned above, and obtaining alcohol treatment since he is more vulnerable to the effects of alcohol after injury.

8. I believe he will be able to cognitively perform his previous job, with the stipulations noted in #7 above.

9. Based on this evaluation, the light duty job requirements that you enclosed are likely within this patient's current abilities and cognitive capacity. I could see him doing this immediately. This, again, should be done on a gradually increasing basis over the course of the next four to six weeks, then re-evaluated for more complex tasks to be added later. All return-to-work activities should be done with observer supervision initially, then periodic checks would be recommended.

I hope these responses address your questions adequately. Please feel free to contact me at 555-0011 if you wish further clarification. Again, thank you for referring a most interesting individual for an evaluation.

Best regards,

Leigh Taylor Fender, Ph.D.
Clinical Neuropsychologist

References

1. Bruce, D., On the origin of the term "neuropsychology." *Neuropsychologia*, 23, 813–814, 1985.
2. Kolb, B. and Whishaw, I.Q., *Fundamentals of Human Neuropsychology*, W. H. Freeman and Company, New York, 1990.
3. Rugg, M.D., Ed., *Cognitive Neuroscience*, The MIT Press, Cambridge, MA, 1997.
4. Pincus, J.H. and Tucker, G.J., *Behavioral Neurology*, Oxford University Press, New York, 1985.
5. Mesulam, M-M., Ed., *Principles of Behavioral Neurology*, F. A. Davis Company, Philadelphia, 1985.
6. Engel, G.L., The clinical application of the biopsychosocial model. *American Journal of Psychiatry*, 137, 535–544, 1980.
7. Paris, J., *Social Factors in the Personality Disorders: A Biopsychosocial Approach to Etiology and Treatment*, Cambridge University Press, Boston, MA, 1996.
8. Kareken, D.A., Judgment pitfalls in estimating premorbid intellectual function. *Archives of Clinical Neuropsychology*, 12, 701–710, 1997.
9. Franzen, M.D., Burgess, E.J., and Smith-Seemiller, L., Methods of estimating premorbid functioning. *Archives of Clinical Neuropsychology*, 12, 711–738, 1997.

10. Williams, J.M., The prediction of premorbid memory ability. *Archives of Clinical Neuropsychology*, 12, 745–756, 1997.
11. Hartlage, L.C., Clinical aspects and issues in assessing premorbid IQ and cognitive function. *Archives of Clinical Neuropsychology*, 12, 763–768, 1997.
12. Reynolds, C.R., Postscripts on premorbid ability estimation: Conceptual addenda and a few words on alternative and conditional approaches. *Archives of Clinical Neuropsychology*, 12, 769–778, 1997.
13. American Psychiatric Association, *Diagnostic and Statistical Manual of Mental Disorders, Fourth Edition*, American Psychiatric Association, Washington, D.C., 1994.
14. Folstein, M.F., Folstein, S.E., and McHugh, P.R., "Mini-Mental State": A practical method for grading the cognitive state of outpatients for the clinician. *Journal of Psychiatric Research*, 12, 189–198, 1975.
15. Hubel, D.H., The brain, in *The Brain*, American Scientific., Inc., W. H. Freeman and Company, New York, 1979, chap 1.
16. Sacks, O., *The Man Who Mistook His Wife for a Hat: and Other Clinical Tales*, Touchstone Books, New York, 1998.
17. Stuss, D.T. and Benson, D.F., *The Frontal Lobes*, Raven Press, New York, 1986.
18. American Psychological Association, Definition of a clinical neuropsychologist. *The Clinical Neuropsychologist*, 3, 22, 1989.

Appendix A: Further reading

The following represents some current resource texts, journals, and websites that provide more in-depth content in the general field of neuropsychology. Neuropsychologists both in academic and applied settings commonly refer to these resources.

Textbooks

Lezak, M.D. (1998). *Neuropsychological Assessment*, Third Edition. New York: Oxford University Press. This textbook likely represents one of the most widely read books in neuropsychology to date. It is commonly used as a required textbook in graduate training programs in neuropsychology as well as being a standard reference text for the practicing neuropsychologist. Now in its third edition, Lezak covers a broad range of neuropsychological tests from a review standpoint, but also provides a discussion of many tests in greater detail. There are excellent sections in the book that cover neuroanatomy and neurological disorders.

Spreen, O. and Strauss, E. (1998). *A Compendium of Neuropsychological Tests: Administration, Norms, and Commentary*, Second Edition. New York: Oxford University Press. In this textbook, Spreen and Strauss have compiled a synopsis of a plethora of currently utilized neuropsychological tests. Each test is described in detail with regard to the history of its development, the particular cognitive or neurobehavioral realms that a test purports to measure, and its reliability and validity. Administration procedures are described and norms are provided from which the clinician may interpret obtained test scores. This second edition also contains further detail on research findings in brain–behavior relationships, developments in cognitive psychology, and in psychological assessment in general. Information about the framework within which neuropsychological assessments are conducted is added to this edition. This book represents another reference text that neuropsychologists employ in their daily practice.

Horton, A.M., Wedding, D., and Webster, J. (Eds.). (1997). *The Neuropsychology Handbook*, Second Edition, *Volume 1: Foundations and Assessment; Volume 2: Treatment Issues and Special Populations*. New York: Springer Publishing Company. This two-volume set contains a wealth of information about the foundations of neuropsychology, its history, relationship of brain structures to behavior, an overview of neurological disorders, and general issues of assessment. The authors also cover topics related to intervention including cognitive retraining, family intervention, and neurobehavioral aspects of brain injury. Special topics concerning pediatric populations, learning disability, HIV/AIDS, toxic exposure, and forensic considerations of neuropsychology are also covered.

Sbordone, R.J. and Long, C.L. (Eds.). (1996). *Ecological Validity of Neuropsychological Testing*, Boca Raton, FL: St. Lucie Press. The relationship between neuropsychological test scores and real-world functioning continues to be a significant issue for academic and practicing neuropsychologists alike. These authors have organized a set of chapters by a range of authors who examine the research and clinical issues that undergird the difficulties in drawing appropriate conclusions from neuropsychological test scores. Directions for developing new instruments that possess better ecological validity are discussed.

Naugle, R.I., Cullum, C.M., and Bigler, E.D. (1998). *Introduction to Clinical Neuropsychology: A Casebook.* Austin, TX: Pro-Ed. The content of this book is introductory in nature and provides the reader an overview of how brain function and neuropsychological functioning of the individual are integrated. This is achieved through the presentation of common neurobehavioral syndromes in their typical form. Case examples are amply used throughout to illustrate these typical neuropsychological presentations of disorders. The combination of quantitative and qualitative approaches to a neuropsychological evaluation is put forth as an effective method of thoroughly examining the patient.

Adams, R.L., Parsons, O.A., Culbertson, J.L., and Nixon, S.J. (Eds.). (1996). *Neuropsychology for Clinical Practice: Etiology, Assessment, and Treatment of Common Neurological Disorders.* American Psychological Association, Washington, D.C. This represents another comprehensive text that covers a broad range of topics and is geared toward the practicing neuropsychologist, yet it is readable by non-neuropsychologists as well. As the title implies, the book is organized by the examination of etiological factors associated with various brain disorders, assessment approaches in neuropsychology, and scientifically based treatment methods for these disorders.

Grant, I. and Adams, K.M. (Eds.). (1996). *Neuropsychological Assessment of Neuropsychiatric Disorders,* Second Edition. New York: Oxford University Press. The editors of this volume have brought together some of the leading researchers in the field of neuropsychology to provide a state-of-the-art compendium of information regarding a range of neuropsychiatric disorders. The book begins with a series of chapters on methods of neuropsychological assessment, covering both fixed and flexible battery approaches. Specific discussion of neuropsychiatric disorders follows and includes chapters on dementia, Tourette's Syndrome, epilepsy, Parkinson's Disease, Huntington's Disease, cerebral vascular disease, hypoxemia, HIV infection, alcoholism, drug abuse, schizophrenia, and traumatic brain injury.

Gronwall, D., Wrightson, P., and Waddell, P. (1998). *Head Injury: The Facts.* New York: Oxford University Press. The authors detail the mechanisms and consequences of brain injury in this highly readable text. This text is not only useful to the clinician, but it can be employed as reading material for family members or others associated with a client having a brain injury.

Levin, H.S., Benton, A.L., Muizelaar, J.P., and Eisenberg, H.M. (Eds.). (1996). *Catastrophic Brain Injury.* New York: Oxford University Press. Severe brain injury is most often associated with somewhat poor functional outcomes, due to the nature of the injury. In this volume, several authors discuss the research findings and reasons for these poor outcomes. Neuropathological findings, national databases, and concomitant medical conditions provide points of reference for describing severe brain injury.

Meier, M.J., Benton, A.L., and Diller, L. (Eds.). (1987). *Neuropsychological Rehabilitation*, New York: Guilford Press. Although this is an older text, many of the chapters continue to have relevance with regard to effective brain injury rehabilitation. The relationship between assessment findings and rehabilitation is explicated by some of the authors. Particular rehabilitation procedures, such as in cognitive remediation, visual perceptual rehabilitation, aphasia therapy, addressing problems with reasoning and problem-solving, and a discussion of psychosocial outcomes appear in this book.

Stringer, A.Y. (1996). *A Guide to Adult Neuropsychological Diagnosis*. Philadelphia, PA: F.A. Davis Company. This author takes a slightly different approach to the presentation of neuropsychological assessment. Various arenas of disorder are covered in exacting detail with descriptions of the cognitive constructs, variances in presentation of a syndrome, etiology, disabling consequences, assessment instruments for constructs, treatment, and case presentation. The book covers disorders of alertness, concentration, stimulus neglect, stimulus imperception, spatial imperception, visual-motor integration, stimulus localization, stimulus recognition, interhemispheric transfer, voluntary cognitive control of movement, oral language, written language, emotional communication, calculation disorders, memory disorders, illusion and hallucination, emotion, and intelligence. This is a comprehensive text that can be used as a reference book for a wide range of disorders.

Heilman, K.M. and Valenstein, E. (1993). *Clinical Neuropsychology*, Third Edition. New York: Oxford University Press. The classic text in neuropsychology covers the major neurobehavioral disorders in detail. Most of the disorders that are covered involve higher level cortical functioning deficits: aphasia, alexia, agraphia, agnosia, apraxia, amnestic dysfunction, and dementia. Methods of diagnosis and treatment are also examined for each of these areas.

Puente, A.E. and McCaffrey, R.J. (Eds.), (1992). *Handbook of Neuropsychological Assessment: A Biopsychosocial Perspective (Critical Issues in Neuropsychology)*. New York: Plenum Press. Although much of what is covered in this text is similar to many other comprehensive texts in neuropsychology, these authors organized the content to take a particular biopsychosocial viewpoint. The interplay of biological, psychological, and social factors is taken into account when discussing brain–behavior relationships.

Reitan, R. and Wolfson, D. (1985). *Neuroanatomy and Neuropathology: A Clinical Guide for Neuropsychologists*. Tucson, AZ: Neuropsychology Press. Although this is an older text and the medical drawings contained within the text are sometimes difficult to follow, the authors are quite articulate in describing essential neurophysiological concepts that relate directly to particular neurological disorders. Normal and abnormal pathologies are discussed for several major neurological conditions.

Reitan, R. (1986). *Traumatic Brain Injury: Pathophysiology and Neuropsychological Evaluation*. Tucson, AZ: Neuropsychology Press. Reitan, R. (1987). *Traumatic Brain Injury: Recovery and Rehabilitation*. Tucson, AZ: Neuropsychology Press. These texts appear as a two-volume set that thoroughly describes the neurophysiology, neuropsychology, and rehabilitation of traumatic brain injury. These are highly readable and well-illustrated texts that can provide a solid foundation of knowledge with particular respect to traumatic brain injury.

Mesulam, M.M. (1985). *Principles of Behavioral Neurology*. Philadelphia, PA: F.A. Davis Company. A closely related field to neuropsychology is behavioral neurology. Composed primarily of neurologists, the field parallels and overlaps a great deal with neuropsychology due to the fact that both fields examine brain–behavior relationships. This text covers in depth the neurophysiology of brain function and dysfunction, and provides a clinical approach to evaluating various neurological conditions. A fine description of neuropsychological testing of older adults appears in this text, and is an example of how behavioral neurology and neuropsychology cover common professional and academic ground.

Kolb, B. and Whishaw, I.Q. (1990). *Fundamentals of Human Neuropsychology*. Third Edition. New York: W. H. Freeman and Company. Understanding basic neuroanatomy and neurophysiology of the brain is foundational to understanding brain–behavior relationships. Kolb and Whishaw's text provides such a foundation for those interested in examining the central nervous system in greater detail. This text is frequently used in graduate training programs as an introductory text to the physiological aspects of brain functioning. It is well-illustrated and easily read by the non-neuropsychologist.

Prigatano, G.P. and Schacter, D.L. (Eds.). (1991). *Awareness of Deficit After Brain Injury: Clinical and Theoretical Issues*. New York: Oxford University Press. Neurobehavioral syndromes complicate the process of brain injury rehabilitation and add another dimension to the process of vocational re-entry for the client with brain injury. These authors describe well what is known as deficit awareness syndromes in a range of brain disorders, including traumatic brain injury. This is a thoughtful volume that not only covers critical research issues but also clearly describes the clinical dilemmas that arise when working with an individual who evidences these problems.

Luria, A.R. (1973). *The Working Brain: An Introduction to Neuropsychology*. New York: Basic Books. Karl Pribam, an internationally known Stanford neuroscientist, articulates the legacy of Aleksandr Luria and the impact he has made upon the field of neuropsychology: "For the past fifty years he has refined clinical observation by devising bedside tests that could be administered to brain-damaged patients and correlated with surgical and pathological reports. Consistently he has shrewdly framed his interpretations of such correlations within the rapidly growing body of knowledge in the neurological and behavioral sciences." Luria pioneered many concepts that were only recently verified by empirical methods owing to the genius of this neuropsychologist. In this book, Luria describes a heuristic for understanding brain–behavior systems, as well as backing his arguments with neurophysiological data, which at that time were still in the early stages of formulation regarding brain–behavior relationships. This book has been considered for a long-time a classical work in a range of fields concerned with brain research and clinical application.

Luria, A.R. and Bruner, J.S. (1987). *The Man with a Shattered World: The History of a Brain Wound*. Boston, MA: Harvard University Press. Part of the brilliance of Luria has been the rare combination of scientific rigor and clinical acumen that is found in this man. This book is an interplay of a person with brain injury telling his story and experience, and Luria's commentary and observations of that individual. This is a moving account of patient and doctor that documents well the phenomenology of brain injury.

Journals

Archives of Clinical Neuropsychology. This publication is the official journal of the National Academy of Neuropsychology and is a blend of relevant clinical research, theoretical articles and reviews of current issues and concepts in neuropsychology.

Journal of the International Neuropsychological Society (INS). As the name implies, this journal is the official publication of the INS. The articles are weighted toward rigorous empirical research in many areas of human neuropsychology. Experimental research is emphasized in this journal.

Neuropsychology. The American Psychological Association publishes a number of journals that correspond to the various professional divisions within APA. This journal is connected with Division 40 of the American Psychological Association and publishes primarily empirical research that relates to clinical neuropsychology.

Neuropsychology Abstracts. This APA journal summarizes in abstract form the current literature in a wide range of topics related to neuropsychology. The journal functions well for those who wish to have a readily available update on the latest published research and ways to access reprints to those articles.

Applied Neuropsychology. This is an international neuropsychology journal with specialists from around the world represented on the editorial board. Assessment issues, neuroimaging studies, empirical and case studies are published in this journal.

Psychological Assessment: A Journal of Consulting and Clinical Psychology. This is another APA journal that broadly covers assessment issues; however, neuropsychological assessment issues often appear in articles that are published in this journal.

Assessment. This is a journal published by the test publisher Psychological Assessment Resources (PAR). Articles that appear within this journal reflect general assessment issues; neuropsychology-oriented issues also appear.

Journal of Head Trauma Rehabilitation. Each issue of this journal is thematic and several articles cover a particular area. Emphasis in this journal is on traumatic brain injury, although other forms of brain injury will appear. There is also an emphasis upon the delivery of rehabilitation services, outcome evaluation, and current issues that relate to the economics of health care delivery systems for brain injury.

Brain Injury. This is an internationally based journal that publishes articles of a theoretical and empirical nature. Although traumatic brain injury is represented heavily, many other types of acquired brain injury appear in articles for this journal. The editorial board represents many of the leaders in the field of brain injury research and rehabilitation.

Archives of Physical Medicine and Rehabilitation. This journal is the official publication of the American Academy of Physical Medicine and Rehabilitation and the American Congress of Rehabilitation Medicine. Articles are primarily empirical in content with the occasional review interspersed across volumes. Traumatic brain injury and other forms of brain injury are covered but not necessarily emphasized in this journal.

Websites

www.nan.drexel.edu. This is the official website for the National Academy of Neuropsychology. Information concerning research, training, and the practice of neuropsychology is found here, and links to other neuropsychology and neurology oriented sites also appear.

www.tbims.org. The National Institute of Disability and Rehabilitation Research (NIDRR) has funded a number of center grants across the country, known as the Traumatic Brain Injury Model Systems grants. These have been awarded to clinical and research centers that track individuals with brain injury from trauma center through acute rehabilitation, post-acute rehabilitation, and community re-entry. This website contains publications generated by the TBI Model Systems, offers linkages to other related websites, and also connects to the Center for Outcome Measurement where one can find technical information regarding outcome measures for brain injury rehabilitation.

www.premier.net/~cogito/neuropsy.html. Neuropsychology Central provides links to a wide range of websites that related to neuropsychology, neurology, and the neurosciences. Other organizations within these fields can be accessed through this site. Geriatric neuropsychology information, neuropsychology software, and training issues are also found here.

www.div40.org. Division 40 (Clinical Neuropsychology) is a part of the American Psychological Association, the latter being the largest professional organization for psychology. Bylaws, announcements, membership, training programs, and the Division 40 newsletter appear at this site. Links to other professional organizations in neuropsychology are also provided.

www.med.ohio-state.edu/ins. The International Neuropsychology Society (INS) is one of the larger international professional bodies in neuropsychology.

www.med.umich.edu/abcn. The American Board of Professional Psychology/American Board of Clinical Neuropsychology is one of two recognized board certification organizations.

www.swets.nl/sps/journals/tcn.html. The Clinical Neuropsychologist is a freestanding journal that represents research, academic, and clinical reports in the field. This is just one example of journals that can be accessed, usually for a cost, on-line. Check also the American Psychological Association's webpage (www.apa.org) that lists all of the major APA journals and provides linkages to the abstracts and tables of contents of many journals. APA also offers its members a flat-rate fee to obtain full text versions of APA journal articles.

www.biomednet.com. After one registers for this website (which at the time of this printing is free of charge), the viewer is able to access MEDLINE, which is a widely utilized journal article search engine for which most major medical, psychiatric, and psychological journals are referenced. The Evaluated MEDLINE search engine keeps a cumulative account of one's past literature searches, and demarcates especially important articles in a particular literature search. Links are provided to the journal that appears in the literature search.

Appendix B: Common neuropsychological tests by general cognitive skill area

Neuropsychological test batteries

Halstead-Reitan neuropsychological test battery

Seven Indexed Tests: Category Test; Tactual Performance Test includes Total Time; Memory; Localization; Seashore Rhythm Test; Speech-Sounds Perception Test; Finger Oscillation Test

Allied Procedures: Grip Strength Test; Reitan-Klove Sensory Perceptual Examination; Lateral Dominance Test; Name Writing Test; Tactual Form Recognition; Test of Visual Fields

Luria-Nebraska neuropsychological test battery

Clinical Scales: Motor Functions; Rhythm; Tactile Functions; Visual Functions; Receptive Speech; Expressive Speech; Writing; Reading; Arithmetic

Localization Scales: Left Frontal; Left Sensorimotor; Left Parietal-Occipital; Left Temporal; Right Frontal; Right Sensorimotor; Right Parietal-Occipital; Right Temporal; Memory; Intellectual Processes; Intermediate Memory

Summary Scales: Pathognomonic; Left Hemisphere; Right Hemisphere; Profile Elevation; Impairment

Cognitive Area	Procedure/Test
Estimates of premorbid or preinjury functioning	Barona Index (for WAIS-R scores); North American Adult Reading Test; Information and Vocabulary Subtests of the Wechsler Adult Intelligence Scale (WAIS-R, WAIS-III); Quick Test of Intelligence
General neuro-psychological functioning	Halstead Impairment Index; Neuropsychological Deficit Scale; Wechsler Adult Intelligence Scale-III: Verbal IQ, Performance IQ, Full Scale IQ; Digit Symbol subtest (WAIS-III); Symbol Digit Modalities Test; Wechsler Memory Scale-III: General Memory Index; WAIS-R as a Neuropsychological Instrument (WAIS-R NI); Mini-Mental State Examination; Neurobehavioral Cognitive Status Examination (Cognistat); Dementia Rating Scale; Stroop Neuropsychological Screening Test; Scales of Cognitive Ability for Traumatic Brain Injury (SCATBI); Brief Test of Head Injury; MicroCog: Assessment of Cognitive Functioning; Quick Neurological Screening Test-2; Severe Impairment Battery; Kaufman Short Neuropsychological Assessment Procedure
Intellectual abilities	Wechsler Adult Intelligence Scale (WAIS-R; WAIS-III); Stanford-Binet Intelligence Test; Quick Test of Intelligence; Shipley Institute of Living Scale; Wonderlic Personnel Test; Raven's Progressive Matrices; Woodcock Tests of Cognitive Ability; Test of Nonverbal Intelligence; Comprehensive Test of Nonverbal Intelligence; Woodcock-Johnson Tests of Cognitive Ability; Kaufman Brief Intelligence Test; Slosson Full-Range Intelligence Test; Beery Picture Vocabulary Test
Academic achievement	Wide Range Achievement Test – 3; Woodcock-Johnson Tests of Achievement; Woodcock Diagnostic Reading Battery; Detroit Tests of Learning Aptitude, 4th Edition; Multidimensional Aptitude Battery
Attention and concentration	Digit Span (WAIS-R/WAIS-III); Arithmetic (WAIS-R; WAIS-III); Working Memory Index (WAIS-III); Working Memory Index (Wechsler Memory Scale-III); Consonant Trigrams Test; Trailmaking Test, Parts A and B; Color Trails Test; Paced Auditory Serial Addition Test; Speech-Sounds Perception Test; Seashore Rhythm Test; Digit Vigilance Test; Stroop Color-Word Test; Letter Cancellation Test; Ruff 2 & 7 Selective Attention Test; Visual Search and Attention Test; Test of Everyday Attention; Brief Test of Attention; Conners' Continuous Performance Test; Test of Variables of Attention; Concentration Endurance Test (d2 Test)

Specific Cognitive Areas and Corresponding Test

Specific Cognitive Areas and Corresponding Test (continued)

Cognitive Area	Procedure/Test
Language processing	Boston Diagnostic Aphasia Battery; Boston Assessment of Severe Aphasia; Multilingual Aphasia Examination, Third Edition; Minnesota Test for Differential Diagnosis of Aphasia; Western Aphasia Battery; Woodcock Language Proficiency Battery – Revised; Neurosensory Center Comprehensive Examination for Aphasia; Controlled Oral Word Association Test; Peabody Picture Vocabulary Test – Revised; Revised Token Test; Reitan-Indiana Aphasia Screening Test
Memory functioning	Wechsler Memory Scale (WMS-R; WMS-III); Memory Assessment Scales; Wide Range Assessment of Memory and Learning; Test of Memory and Learning; Rivermead Behavioural Memory Test; California Verbal Learning Test; Rey Auditory Verbal Learning Test; Buschke Selective Reminding Test; Rey-Osterrieth Complex Figure Test (and Taylor alternate version); Rey Complex Figure Test and Recognition Trial; Rey Visual Design Learning Test; Benton Visual Retention Test; Tactual Performance Test (Memory; Location); Continuous Visual Memory Test; Sentence Repetition Test; Fuld Object-Memory Evaluation
Speed of cognitive processing	Trailmaking Test, Parts A and B; Tactual Performance Test (Total Time); Processing Speed Index (WAIS-III); Speed and Capacity of Language-Processing Test; Symbol Digit Modalities Test
Visuospatial and perceptual-motor integration abilities	Perceptual Organization Index (WAIS-III); Rey-Osterrieth Complex Figure Test; Hooper Visual Organization Test; Clock Drawing Test; Bicycle Drawing Test; Benton Visual Retention Test; Judgment of Line Orientation; Visual Form Discrimination Test; Tactile Form Perception Test; Three-Dimensional Block Construction Test; Facial Recognition Test; Right-Left Orientation Test; Tactual Form Recognition Test (Halstead-Reitan); Embedded Figures Test
Sensory, tactile, and motor functioning	Tactual Performance Test (Total Time); Tactile Form Perception; Tactile Form Recognition; Finger Localization (Benton); Reitan-Klove Sensory Perceptual Examination; Finger Oscillation Test (Finger Tapping Test); Hand Dynamometer Test; Grooved Pegboard Test; Purdue Pegboard Test; Minnesota Manual Dexterity Test

Specific Cognitive Areas and Corresponding Test (continued)

Cognitive Area	Procedure/Test
Complex problem-solving, adaptive reasoning, novel problem-solving; executive functioning	Category Test; Wisconsin Card Sorting Test; Tactual Performance Test; Trailmaking Test, Part B; Behavioural Assessment of the Dysexecutive Syndrome; Ruff Figural Fluency Test; Tower of London Test; Cookie Theft Picture Test (Boston Diagnostic Aphasia Examination)
Psychological assessment and personality inventories	Minnesota Multiphasic Personality Inventory-2; Millon Clinical Multiaxial Inventory-III; Millon Behavioral Health Inventory; Millon Inventory of Personality Styles; NEO Personality Inventory – Revised; 16 Personality Factor Inventory, Fifth Edition; Clinical Analysis Questionnaire (Cattell); Interpersonal Adjective Checklist ; Personality Assessment Inventory (Morey); Myers-Briggs Personality Indicators
Psychosocial assessment	Sickness Impact Profile; Coping Responses Inventory (Moos); Life Stressors and Social Resources Inventory (Moos); Family Environment Scale; Family Assessment Device; Psychosocial Pain Inventory (Heaton)
Mood assessment	Beck Depression Inventory-II; Beck Anxiety Scale; Beck Hopelessness Scale; Beck Scale for Suicide Ideation; Hamilton Depression Rating Scale; Hamilton Depression Inventory; Zung Depression Scale; Center for Epidemiological Studies Depression Scale; Geriatric Depression Scale; State-Trait Anxiety Inventory; State-Trait Anger Expression Inventory; State-Trait-Depression Adjective Check Lists

Appendix C: Glossary of common terms in neuropsychology*

Abstract thinking: A style of thinking in which language is interpreted conceptually. The ability to reason and to solve problems.

Abulia: Loss or deficit in initiative or drive; inability to sustain speech output and narrative.

Acalculia: The inability to perform problems of arithmetic.

Acuity: Sharpness or quality of a sensation.

Affect: Range and appropriateness of emotional responses; the visual presentation of emotion; can be described as restricted, blunt, flat, appropriate, or labile.

Agnosia: Failure to recognize familiar objects even though the sensory mechanism is intact.

Agraphia: Inability to express thoughts in writing.

Alexia: Inability to read.

Amnesia: Lack of memory about events occurring during a particular period of time. See also retrograde amnesia, post-traumatic amnesia, and anterograde amnesia.

Aneurysm: A balloon-like deformity in the wall of a blood vessel. This wall weakens as the balloon grows larger, and may eventually burst, causing a hemorrhage.

Anhedonia: Loss of feeling of pleasure; inability to experience pleasure or engage in pleasant activities.

Anomia: Inability to recall names of objects. Such patients can often speak fluently, but have to use other words to describe familiar objects.

Anosognosia: Limited or shallow awareness of oneself. Usually in brain injury it refers to a limited ability to recognize one's deficits in cognitive and behavioral abilities.

Anosmia: Loss of the sense of smell.

Anoxia: A lack of oxygen. Cells of the brain need oxygen to stay alive. When blood flow to the brain is reduced or when oxygen in the blood is too low, brain cells are damaged.

Anterograde amnesia: Inability to consolidate information about ongoing events. Sometimes referred to as recent memory deficit.

Anticonvulsant: Medication used to decrease the possibility of a seizure. These include Dilantin, Tegretol, Phenobarbital, Depakote and Neurontin among others.

Apathy: A general lack of interest or concern.

---

* Taken largely and primarily from the *Brain Injury Glossary*, The Institute for Rehabilitation and Research (TIRR), Traumatic Brain Injury Model System Research Program, Texas Medical Center, 1333 Moursund Avenue, Houston, Texas 77030.

Aphasia: Loss of the ability to express oneself and/or to understand language. Caused by damage to brain cells rather than deficits in motor speech abilities or hearing organs.

Aphasia, expressive: Inability to find or formulate the words to express oneself even though knowing what one wants to say.

Aphasia, global: Severely limited residual ability to communicate with others. Includes both expressive and receptive aphasia.

Aphasia, nonfluent: Characterized by awkward articulation, limited vocabulary, hesitant, slow speech output, restricted use of grammatical forms, and a relative preservation of auditory comprehension.

Aphasia, receptive: Problems in understanding what others attempt to communicate.

Aphemia: The isolated loss of the ability to articulate words without loss of the ability to write or comprehend spoken language.

Apraxia: Inability to carry out a complex or skilled movement not due to paralysis, sensory changes, or deficiencies in understanding.

Apraxia, constructional: Inability to assemble, build, draw or copy accurately; not due to apraxia of single movements. Many patients will be dyspraxic, meaning a decreased ability for construction praxis.

Apraxia, ideomotor: Deficit in the execution of a movement due to inability to access the instructions to muscles stored by previous motor experience.

Arteriovenous malformation: An abnormal "tangle" of blood vessels present from birth that may be prone to bleeding

Asomatognosia: Loss of knowledge or awareness about one's own body or condition.

Astereognosia: Inability to recognize things by touch.

Ataxia: A problem of muscle coordination not due to apraxia, weakness, rigidity, spasticity, or sensory loss. Caused by lesion of the cerebellum or basal ganglia. Can interfere with a person's ability to walk, talk, eat, and to perform other self-care tasks.

Attention/concentration: Refers to the person's ability to attend and then sustain focus on a task, in the face of other stimuli in the environment.

Augmentive communication: An area of the clinical practice of speech and language pathology in which attempts are made to compensate, enhance, or remove obstacles to expressive communication.

Autotopagnosia: Inability to localize, names, or orient correctly different parts of the body.

Balint's syndrome: Visual fixation of cortical origin with deficits in visual attention, associated with perseverative eye movements.

Bell's palsy: Paralysis of the face due to facial nerve injury, associated with distortion in facial expression and appearance.

Bilateral: Pertaining to both right and left sides.

Bradykinesia: Abnormal slowing of body movement; slowed physical and mental responses to stimuli.

Brain injury, mild: Sometimes also referred to as minor traumatic brain injury; people who sustain this level of injury: (1) had sustained some disruption of neurologic function due to damage to brain tissue or structures. Such damage is often difficult to detect using CT Scans, may sometimes be seen on MRI Scans, may result in abnormalities in EEG; (2) had sustained loss of consciousness of less than 30 minutes — usually a matter of a few minutes; (3) have obtained a Glasgow Coma Scale score of 13 to 15; and 4) have characteristic post-head trauma symptoms in the physical, cognitive, and behavioral realms.

Brain injury, moderate: Such individuals usually: (1) have had documented evidence of brain tissue or structural damage on CT, MRI, EEG, or other neurological assessment method; (2) obtain Glasgow Coma Scale scores of between 9 and 12; and (3) often have significant cognitive, physical, and behavioral impairments that interfere with long-term vocational goals and community/home functioning.

Brain injury, severe: Such individuals: (1) have documented evidence of brain tissue or structural damage; (2) obtain Glasgow Coma Scale score of 8 or less; and (3) have significant and often pervasive physical, cognitive, and behavioral impairments that greatly interfere with long-term vocational goals and community/home functioning.

Buccofacial apraxia: Oral apraxia characterized by an inability to execute skilled movements in the face and in speech mechanisms, usually with normal comprehension abilities.

Capgras syndrome: Misidentification of family members, friends, and other loved ones as not the "real" person but rather the patient considers them as imposters. This is an example of a disconnection syndrome between limbic structures and higher cortical areas of the brain.

Cataplexy: A sudden loss of muscle tone that results from exaggerated emotional output such as in excessive laughter or anger. Can be associated with narcolepsy.

Cerebral hemorrhage: Massive bleeding into brain tissue, often caused by hypertension.

Cerebral infarct: When the blood supply is reduced below a critical level and the brain tissue in that region dies. Commonly referred to as a stroke.

Cerebrospinal fluid (CSF): A liquid which fills the ventricles of the brain and surrounds the brain and spinal cord.

Chorea: Involuntary, complex, and arrhythmic movements that appear rapid, jerky, and occur with variance in speed and regularity; can be caused by damage to putamen and striatum.

Clonus: A sustained series of rhythmic jerks following quick stretch of a muscle.

Cognition: The conscious process of knowing or being aware of thoughts or perceptions, including understanding, remembering, and reasoning.

Coma: A state of unconsciousness from which the patient cannot be aroused, even by significant stimulation. Not to be confused with a sleeping state.

Concrete thinking: A style of thinking in which the individual sees each situation as unique and is unable to generalize from the similarities between situations. Thinking in which language is interpreted literally.

Concussion: A transient change in neurologic function due to a mechanical force being applied to the head. This usually causes brief loss of consciousness or altered ability to think and be oriented.

Confabulation: Verbalizations about people, places, and/or events with no basis in reality. The patient appears to "fill in the gaps" in memory with plausible facts. The patient is not aware of the unreality of such verbalizations.

Confusion: A state in which a person is bewildered, perplexed, or unable to self-orient.

Consciousness: The state of awareness of the self and the environment.

Continence: The ability to control urination and bowel movements.

Contractures: Loss of range of motion in a joint due to abnormal shortening of soft tissues.

Contralateral: Opposite side.

Contrecoup: Bruising of the brain tissue on the side opposite from which a blow was struck.

Contusion: A bruise. The result of a blow to the head which bruises brain tissue.

Cortex: The convoluted outer layer of brain gray matter, composed of nerve cell bodies; the system of cortical sulci and gyri that compose the gray matter area of the brain.

Cortical blindness: Loss of vision resulting from a lesion in the primary visual areas of the occipital lobe.

Coup damage: Damage to the brain at the point of impact.

Decerebrate posturing: Exaggerated posture of extension as a result of a lesion to the prepontine area of the brain stem, which is rarely seen.

Decorticate posturing: Exaggerated posture of upper extremity flexion and lower extremity extension as a result of a lesion to the mesencephalon or above that level.

Decubitus ulcer: Pressure area, bed sore, skin opening, skin breakdown. A discolored or open area of skin damage caused by pressure. Common areas most prone to breakdown are buttocks or backside, hips, shoulder blades, heels, ankles and elbows.

Degenerative disorders: These include the progressive dementias such as Alzheimer's Disease, Pick's Disease, Parkinson's Disease, multi-infarct dementia, Huntington's Disease and alcoholic dementia.

Déjà vu: From the French "seen before." The subjective sensation that a situation being experienced for the first time has been experienced before. Often associated with psychomotor seizures.

Dementia: Disturbances of memory and other higher cortical functioning that are severe enough to disrupt social or occupational functioning. This is in the absence of clouding of consciousness or delirium states.

Diadochokinesia: The function of ceasing one motor output impulse and substituting a diametrically opposite impulse.

Diffuse axonal injury: A shearing injury of large nerve fibers in many areas of the brain due to an impact to the head of significant force. Rotational forces also can produce such lesions. This phenomena is observable primarily by microscopic inspection of brain tissue.

Diplopia: Seeing two images of a single object; double vision.

Discrimination, auditory: The ability to differentiate and recognize sounds.

Discrimination, sensory: A process requiring differentiation of two or more stimuli.

Discrimination, tactile: The ability to identify and distinguish between objects and stimuli solely through touch.

Discrimination, visual: The differentiation of items using sight.

Disinhibition: Inability to suppress (inhibit) impulsive behavior and emotions. This often results from damage to the frontal system and occurs in disconnection syndromes.

Disorientation: Inability or deficits in knowing where you are, who you are, or the current date. Being disoriented "times three" means not knowing person, place, or time.

Disposition: Plans for where the person will live after discharge from the hospital or facility.

Distal: Far from the point of attachment.

Dysarthria: Difficulty forming words or speaking them because of weakness of muscles used in speech. Speech is characterized by slurred imprecise articulation. Tongue movements are usually labored and the rate of speaking may be very slow. Voice quality may be abnormal, usually excessively nasal; volume may be weak; drooling may occur. Dysarthria may accompany aphasia or occur alone.

Dysfluency: Impairment in the ability to generate words upon confrontation; stammering and stuttering are often present.

Dyslexia: Specific developmental learning disorder that is present in childhood, often with children who have normal levels of intellectual functioning, but have unusual difficulties in learning to read; reversal of letters and numbers is associated with this condition.

Dysmetria: Inability to stop a movement at the desired point; also known as past-pointing.

Dysphagia: A swallowing disorder characterized by difficulty in oral preparation for the swallow, or in moving material from the mouth to the stomach. This includes problems with positioning food in the mouth.

Echolalia: Imitation of sounds or words without comprehension. This is a normal stage of language development in infants, but is abnormal in adults.

Edema: Collection of fluid in the tissue causing swelling. Brain edema is a condition that can occur shortly after an injury to brain tissue.

Electrocardiogram (EKG): A record of the electrical activity of the heart, produced by recording devices placed on the chest. It is used routinely in the intensive care unit.

Electroencephalography: A procedure that uses electrodes on the scalp to record electrical activity of the brain. Used for detection of seizure disorders, level of coma, and "brain death." EEGs are often conducted under conditions of quiet wakefulness, sleep, hyperventilation, and photic stimulation conditions.

Embolism: The sudden blocking of an artery or a vein by a blood clot, bubble of air, deposit of oil or fat, or small mass of cells deposited by the blood flow.

Emotional liability: Exhibition of rapid and dramatic changes in emotional state (laughing, crying, anger) without apparent reason.

Encephalitis: Inflammation or abscesses that occur within the central nervous system, caused by infection from virus, bacteria, fungi, or parasitic infestations.

Endotracheal tube: A tube that serves as an artificial airway and is inserted through the patient's mouth or nose. It passes through the throat and into the air passages to help breathing. To do this, it must also pass through the patient's vocal cords. The patient cannot speak when this tube is in place. This tube is connected to a respirator.

Equilibrium: Evoked Polential: Normal balance reactions and postures. Registration of the electrical response of brain cells as detected by electrodes placed on the surface of the head at various places. The evoked potential is elicited by a specific stimulus applied to the visual, auditory, or other sensory receptors of the body. Evoked potentials are used to diagnose a wide variety of central nervous system disorders.

Evoked potentials, brain stem: Auditory brain stem responses provoked by discrete sounds delivered to the ears through headphones. These sound waves are converted to nerve impulses by receptors in the ear. A device is used to test whether the brain stem has received the signals.

Extrapyramidal symptoms: Disorders that arise as side-effects of several different types of antipsychotic medications, neurological disease, and other causes. These symptoms include disruption of movement and symptoms of tardive dyskinesia.

Field Defects: Areas of blindness within the visual field. Depending upon the lesion location, partial or complete blindness of the visual field can result.

Finger agnosia: Inability to identify the fingers, may arise from lesions to either cerebral hemisphere.

Flexion: Bending a joint.

Focal: Restricted to one region (as opposed to diffuse).

Foley catheter: This is a tube inserted into the urinary tract and into the bladder for drainage of urine. The urine flows through the tube and collects into an external plastic bag.

GI tube: A tube inserted through a surgical opening into the stomach. It is used to introduce liquids, food, or medication into the stomach when the patient is unable to take these substances orally.

Glasgow coma scale: A standardized rating system used to categorize the depth of coma and, therefore, brain injury severity. The rating is based upon best eye-opening response, best verbal response, and best motor response. Scores range from a low of 3 to a high of 15. Persons who are considered to have a "mild" brain injury score between 13 to 15. "Moderate" brain injury are scores of 9 to 12; while in the "severe" category, patients obtain scores of 8 and below.

Graphesthesia: Impairment in the ability to identify numbers or letters that are traced on the skin with a blunt ended object (e.g., erasure head of a pencil).

Gray Matter: Refers to the nerve cell bodies which form the brain's content.

Handedness: This refers to the cerebral dominance of the individual. Cerebral Dominance for language and handedness are highly correlated and influenced by genetic transmission.

Head Injury: Usually synonymous with traumatic brain injury.

Hematoma: The collection of blood in tissues or a space following rupture of a blood vessel. After traumatic brain injury, hematomas can occur throughout the brain, or in different spaces including the epidural space, subdural space, or can occur within the cerebrum itself. If the collection of blood is large enough, and is judged to be removable, a hematoma may by evacuated by neurosurgical procedures.

Hemianopsia: Visual field cut. Blindness for one-half or one-quarter of the field of vision. This most frequently involves the right or left half of each eye.

Hemiparesis: Weakness of one side of the body.

Hemiplegia: Paralysis of one side of the body as a result of injury to neurons carrying signals to muscles from the motor areas of the brain.

Hemorrhage: Bleeding that occurs following damage to blood vessels. Bleeding may occur within the brain when blood vessels in the brain are damaged.

Homonymous hemianopsia: Impairment in vision or blindness in the right or left halves of the visual field of both eyes.

Hydrocephalus: Enlargement of fluid-filled cavities in the brain, not due to brain atrophy.

Hypoxemia: Deficient oxygenation of the blood, also known as hypoxia.

ICP: Intracranial pressure. This is often monitored in the intensive care unit and provides information about the need to relieve the pressure if it should rise to critical levels.

Imperception: Failure to perceive stimulation on one side of the body when both sides are being stimulated simultaneously. It is not due to a primary sensory deficit such as deafness or blindness, but is due more to an attentional deficit.

Impersistence: Impairment in the ability to maintain a motor action such as holding one's tongue out or standing on one foot.

Impulse control: Refers to the patient's inability to withhold inappropriate verbal or motor responses while completing a task. It refers to acting or speaking without first considering the consequences.

Incontinence: Inability to control bowel and bladder functions.

Incoordination: A problem with coordination in moving parts of the body, resulting from dysfunction of the nervous system rather than weakness of muscles.

Infarct: An area of dead or dying tissue, often in the cortex. This arises out of an obstruction of the blood vessels that normally serve a particular cortical region.

Insult: Something that causes injury. In referring to an intracranial insult, this refers to a mechanism by which the brain is injured. This includes hematomas (intraparenchymal and extraparenchymal), elevations of intracranial pressure (ICP), brain swelling, edema, and vasospasm.

Intelligence quotient: A measure of general intelligence obtained by testing. It consists of either a ratio of mental age to chronological age or a score of deviation from an expected test performance by age.

Intracerebral: Within the cerebral hemisphere.

Ipsilateral: Same side of the body.

Ischemia: A severe reduction in the supply of blood to body tissues.

Jamais vu: From the French "never seen." The subjective sensation that familiar surroundings are strange or are being experienced for the first time.

Kinesthesia: The sensory awareness of body parts as they move.

Laceration: A ragged tear.

Laconic speech: Speech output characterized by pauses between verbalizations; difficulty in sustaining conversation output and narrative.

Latency of response: The amount of time it takes a person to respond after the stimulus has been presented.

Lateral: Away from the middle portion or midline; opposite of medial.

Laterality: Relating to the degree to which certain functions are localized to the right or left cerebral hemisphere. Laterality is relative since both hemispheres play a role in most behaviors.

Lethargic: Awakens with stimulation; drowsy but awake.

Locked-in syndrome: Paralysis of all muscles in the body, except eye-movement. It occurs with the inability to communicate with others, except through available eye movements. This arises secondary to lesions in the medulla.

Medial: Pertaining to the middle portion of a structure.

Memory, auditory/visual: Auditory memory is the ability to recall numbers, lists of words, sentences, or paragraphs presented orally. Visual memory requires input of information through the visuoperceptual channels. It refers to the ability to recall text, figures, maps, and photographs.

Memory, delayed: The ability to recall information several minutes following presentation. There is no particular specification of the required time interval; typically it is 10 to 30 minutes.

Memory, episodic: Memory for ongoing events in a person's life. More easily impaired than semantic memory, perhaps because rehearsal or repetition tends to be minimal.

Memory, immediate: The ability to recall numbers, pictures, or words immediately following presentation. Patients with immediate memory problems have difficulty learning new tasks because they cannot remember instructions. This relies upon attention and concentration.

Memory, learning: Acquisition of new information determined by the extent to which an individual benefits from repetition, rehearsal, or practice.

Memory, long-term: In neuropsychological testing, this refers to recall 30 minutes or longer after presentation. It requires storage and retrieval of information that exceeds the limit of an immediate period. Long-term memory can often refer to stored information over many years, or over-learned material such as date of birth, childhood memories, home telephone number, etc.

Memory, recall: Ability to retrieve information without renewed exposure to the stimulus.

Memory, recognition: Ability to retrieve information when a familiar stimulus is presented.

Memory, remote: Information an individual correctly recalls from the distant past. There is no specific requirement for the amount of elapsed time, but it is typically more than six months to a year.

Memory, semantic: Memory for facts, usually learned through repetition.

Memory, short-term: Primary or "working" memory, that is, a limited capacity system that holds up to seven chunks of information (plus or minus two) over periods of 30 seconds to several minutes. Often called "recent" memory.

Microcephaly: Development of the brain is rudimentary and this will result in the person having a low level of intelligence.

Mobility: Ability of an individual to move within and interact with the environment. This usually involves utilization of public and/or private transportation.

Mood: Refers to the emotional tone of the patient. Often relates to the subjective experience of the patient with regard to emotion. Includes dysphoric, elevated, euthymic, expansive, irritable and euphoric states.

Motor: Pertaining to movement.

Motor control: Regulation of the timing and amount of contraction of body muscles to produce smooth and coordinated movement. The regulation is carried out by the nervous system's operation.

Motor control, fine: Delicate, intricate movements as in writing or playing a piano.

Motor control, gross: Large, strong movements as in chopping wood or walking.

Motor lag: A prolonged delay between stimulus and initiation of motor response.

Motor planning: Action formulated in the mind before attempting to perform.

Muscle tone: Used in clinical practice to describe the muscle's resistance to being stretched. When the peripheral nerve to a muscle is severed, the muscle becomes flaccid. When nerve fibers in the brain or spinal cord are damaged, the balance between facilitation and inhibition of muscle tone is disturbed. The tone of some muscles may become increased and they resist being stretched -- a condition called hypertonicity or spasticity.

Myasthenia gravis: The patient presents with marked muscle weakness and paralysis; early symptoms include double vision (diplopia) and ptosis (drooping eyelid).

Nasogastric tube (NG tube): A tube which passes through the patient's nose and throat and ends in the patient's stomach.

Neologism: Nonsense or made-up word used when speaking. The person often does not realize that the word makes no sense.

Non-ambulatory: Not able to walk, or unable to walk safely without assistance.

Non-purposeful movement: Movement that a person may make which has no apparent goal.

Nystagmus: Involuntary horizontal, vertical, or rotary movement of the eyeballs.

Obtunded: Mental blunting; mild to moderate reduction in alertness. Usually the person shows very little variation in facial movement or expression.

Occlusion: The mechanics of closure or state of being closed; an obstruction; often relates to impairments in blood flow.

Orientation: An awareness of one's environment and/or situation, and the ability to use this information appropriately in a functional setting.

Orientation, left-right: The ability to discriminate between left and right body parts for oneself and on others, as well as the ability to discriminate between left and right within the environment.

Orientation, personal: General knowledge related to oneself including information regarding date of birth, age, name, and location of home.

Orientation, situational: The ability to accurately describe present circumstances.

Orientation, temporal: Knowledge of the current date, day, month, and year. Includes knowledge of facts related to time of day.

Orthosis: Splint or brace designed to improve function or provide stability.

Palsy: Paralysis.

Paraparesis: Weakness of the lower limbs.

Paraphasic error: Substitution of an incorrect sound (e.g., tree for free) or related word (e.g., chair for bed).

Paraplegia: Paralysis of the legs, from the waist down.

Parapnaisias: Use of incorrect words or word combinations.

Pathognomonic: Specifically related to or characteristic of a disease or disorder.

Perception: The ability to make sense of what one sees, hears, feels, tastes, or smells. Perceptual losses are often very subtle, and the patient and/or family may be unaware of such problems.

Perceptual-motor: Interaction of the perceptual abilities with motor abilities.

Perseveration: Refers to the inappropriate persistence of a response in a current task that may have been appropriate for a former task. Perseverations may be verbal or motoric.

Persistent vegetative state (PVS): A condition in which the patient utters no words and does not follow commands or make any response that is meaningful. The transition of a person who remains unconscious from a state of "coma" to one of being in a "vegetative state" reflects subtle changes over a period of several months from a condition of no response to the internal or external environment (except reflexively) to a state of wakefulness but with no indication of awareness (cortical function). A patient in this state may have a range of biological responses at the subcortical level, such as eye opening (with sleep and wake rhythms) and sometimes the ability to follow with one's eyes.

Phonation: The production of sound by means of vocal cord vibration.

Physiatrist: A physician (M.D.) who specializes in physical medicine and rehabilitation. A physiatrist is an expert in neurologic rehabilitation, trained to diagnose and treat disabling conditions.

Plasticity: Transfer of function from damaged to undamaged brain tissue.

Post-traumatic amnesia: A period of hours, days, or weeks after a brain injury when the patient exhibits a loss of moment-to-moment memory. The patient is unable to store new information and, therefore, has a decreased ability to learn. Patients often report that they have little to no recall of events during the period of post-traumatic amnesia.

Praxis: Motor output and integration in complex learned movements.

Premorbid functioning: Characteristics of an individual present before the disease or injury occurred.

Problem-solving: Ability of the individual to bring cognitive processes to the consideration of how to accomplish a task.

Prognosis: The prospect for recovery from a disease or injury as indicated by the nature and symptoms of the case.

Proprioception: Sensory awareness of body part positions with or without movement.

Prosody: The inflections or intonations of speech.

Prosthesis: An artificial substitute for a missing body part, such as an arm or leg, eye or tooth, used for both functional and cosmetic reasons.

Proximal: Next to, or nearest, the point of attachment.

Psychometrist: A person with a bachelor's or master's degree and training in the administration of psychological and neuropsychological tests. These individuals will administer batteries of tests in a standardized fashion and score test results under the guidance of a psychologist or neuropsychologist.

Psychosocial functioning: Refers to the individual's adjustment to the injury and resulting disability, and one's ability to relate to others. Includes a person's coping style in relation to the injury or illness, social support utilization, and emotional status.

Ptosis: Drooping of a body part, such as the upper eyelid, from paralysis, or drooping of visceral organs from weakness of the abdominal muscles.

Quadriparesis: Weakness of all four limbs.

Quadriplegia: Paralysis of all four limbs.

Range of motion: Refers to movement of a joint. This is important to prevent contractures.

Range of motion, active: The muscles around the joint do the work to move it.

Range of motion, passive: Movement of a joint by means other than contraction of the muscles around that joint (e.g., someone else moves the joint).

Reasoning, concrete: Involves the ability to understand the literal meaning of a phrase.

Reasoning, generalization: The ability to take information, rules, and strategies learned about one situation and apply them appropriately to other, similar situations.

Reasoning, sequential: The ability to organize information or objects according to specified rules, or the ability to arrange information or objects in a logical, progressive manner. Nearly every activity, including work and leisure tasks, requires sequencing.

Recall: The process of remembering and retrieval from memory storage.

Recent memory deficit: See anterograde amnesia.

Reduplication: Distortion of memory recall of geographic locations.

Retrograde amnesia: Inability to recall events prior to the accident; may be a specific span of time or type of information.

Rostral: Toward the head; up or above.

Scanning: The active search of the environment for information; usually refers to "visual scanning" which is a skill used in reading, driving, and many daily activities.

Scotoma: An area of blindness of varying size within the visual fields.

Seizure: An uncontrolled discharge of electrical activity in nerve cells that may spread to other nearby cells in the brain. It usually lasts only a few minutes. It may be associated with loss of consciousness, convulsions, loss of bowel and bladder control, and tremors. May also cause disoriented actions or other behavioral change—symptoms vary with seizure type.

Sensorimotor: Refers to all aspects of movement and sensation and the interaction of the two.

Sequencing: Reading, listening, expressing thoughts, describing events, or contracting muscles in an orderly and meaningful manner.

Shunt: A procedure to draw off excessive fluid in the brain. A surgically placed polythene cannula (tube) running from the ventricles which deposits fluid into the abdominal cavity, heart, or large veins of the neck.

Skull fracture: The breaking of the bone surrounding the brain. A depressed skull fracture is one in which the broken bone exerts pressure on the brain.

Spasticity: An involuntary increase in muscle tone (tension) that occurs following injury to the brain or spinal cord, causing the muscles to resist being moved. Characteristics may include an increase in deep tendon reflexes, resistance to passive stretch, clasp knife phenomenon, and clonus.

Spatial ability: Ability to perceive the construction of an object in both two and three dimensions. Spatial ability is composed of four components: the ability to perceive a static figure in different positions, the ability to interpret and duplicate the movements between various parts of a figure, the ability to perceive the relationship between object and a person's own body sphere, and the ability to interpret the person's body as an object in space.

Spontaneous recovery: The recovery which occurs as damage to body tissues heal. This type of recovery occurs with or without rehabilitation, and it is very difficult to know how much improvement is spontaneous and how much is due to rehabilitative interventions.

Status epilepticus: Continuous seizures; may produce permanent brain damage. After five minutes of a major motor seizure, medical aid should be called.

Stereognosis: Ability to recognize objects through tactile senses.

Strabismus: Misalignment of the eyes.

Stroke: See cerebral infarct.

Stupor: Deep sleep; is unresponsive but person can be awakened with repeated, noxious stimulation. Awareness is depressed but present.

Subdural: Beneath the dura (tough membrane) covering the brain and spinal cord.

Supine: Lying on one's back.

Syncope: A period of time when the patient loses consciousness accompanied by weakness in smooth muscles, and inability to stand upright.

Tactile discrimination: The ability to differentiate information received through the sense of touch. Sharp/dull discrimination — ability to distinguish between sharp and dull stimuli; two-point discrimination — the ability to recognize two points applied to the skin simultaneously as distinct from one single point.

Tardive dyskinesia: Deficits in voluntary motor output and movement, characterized by incomplete or intermittent movement output, often associated with long-term antipsychotic medication use.

Telegraphic speech: Speech that sounds like a telegram. Only the main words of a sentence (nouns, verbs) are present; the small words (ifs, ands, buts) are missing. This type of speech often gets the message across.

Thrombus: Blood clot.

Tonic-clonic seizure: Formerly called "Grand mal" seizure involving generalized rigidity of the body (tonic stage) and then generalized convulsions (clonic stage).

Tracking, visual: Visually following an object as it moves through space.

Transfer: Moving one's body between wheelchair and bed, toilet, mat, or car with or without the assistance of another person.

Transient ischemic attacks (TIAs): Temporary interference of the blood supply to the brain. Although the symptoms may last from a few minutes to hours, no identifiable, permanent, neurological damage results.

Tremor, intention: Coarse, rhythmical movements of a body part that become intensified the harder one tries to control them.

Tremor, resting: Rhythmical movements present at rest and may be diminished during voluntary movement.

Unilateral: Pertaining to only one side.

Unilateral neglect: Paying little or no attention to things on one side of the body. This usually occurs on the side opposite from the location of the injury to the brain because nerve fibers from the brain typically cross before innervating body structures. In extreme cases, the patient may not bathe, dress, or acknowledge one side of the body.

Ventral: Toward the base of the brain.

Ventricles, brain: Four natural cavities in the brain that are filled with cerebrospinal fluid. The outline of one or more of these cavities may change when a space-occupying lesion (hemorrhage, tumor) has developed in a lobe of the brain.

Verbal fluency: The ability to produce words.

Vestibular: Pertaining to the vestibular system in the middle ear and the brain that senses movements of the head. Disorders of the vestibular system can lead to dizziness, poor regulation of postural muscle tone, and inability to detect quick movements of the head.

Visual agnosia: Impairment in the recognition of objects despite intact visual input.

Visual field defect: Inability to see objects located in a specific region of the field of view ordinarily received by each eye. Often the blind region includes everything in the right half or left half of the visual field.

Visual imagery: The use of mental pictures to aid in recall.

Visual perception: The ability to recognize and discriminate between visual stimuli and to interpret these stimuli through association with earlier experiences. For example, to separate a figure from a background, to synthesize the contents of a picture, and to interpret the invariability of an object which is seen from different directions.

White matter: The area within the cerebral cortex that consists of axons. These axons are connected to the nerve cells (which make up the gray matter).

chapter two

Counseling interactions for clients with traumatic brain injury

Keith D. Cicerone, Ph.D. and Robert T. Fraser, Ph.D., C.R.C.

Introduction

Traumatic brain injury represents a tremendous obstacle to effective functioning for clients, which is very often expressed through their difficulty and frustration around the issue of work return. This is not surprising in our culture and society, since the inability to return to work carries both social and economic costs, and notions of *recovery of function* and *being normal* are associated (rightly and wrongly) with return to work. Not only clients and family members, but also rehabilitation therapists, counselors, and funding agencies often see return as the signpost of successful rehabilitation and recovery after traumatic brain injury. Price and Baumann (1990)[1] point out that working is often considered the key to normalization after a traumatic brain injury, since many of these clients have already established normal developmental milestones including personal and career decisions.

The other paramount concern is the ability to function independently relative to activities of daily living and socialization. If individuals can't work, can they maintain a home and engage in the social fabric of the community through organizational activity, use of recreational resources, and volunteering?

Traumatic injury interferes with a lifelong process through which a person was establishing a personal identity and social role. The injury, and particularly the inability to work, thereby disrupts the individual's sense of purpose, productivity and self-worth. The inability to work may have far-reaching consequences for a person's capacity in autonomous functioning. For this reason, the central concern of the counseling process can be seen as one of assisting a person to re-establish a satisfactory level of *personal and functional sufficiency*. We use the concept of personal sufficiency to refer to a person's ability to function and achieve goals with various levels of assistance or reliance on others, and with the aim of acknowledging a need for interdependence.

With respect to vocational counseling, an emphasis may be placed on fostering the client's ability to make choices, facilitating a sense of self-determination, and providing him with the appropriate resources. This can often involve allowing the client to make decisions with which the therapist or counselor does not agree, or which in fact appear to be unrealistic. Unlike the client with a history of developmental disability, the traumatically injured client with severe brain injury is forced to re-align expectancies for future functioning despite having a personal history of career decisions and achievement. Clients will often respond negatively to the suggestion that they will be unable to attain 100% of their pre-injury status, and cling stubbornly to their aspirations even when faced with repeated, objective evidence to the contrary. The emotional responses to this confrontation can include depression, catastrophic anxiety, minimization of deficits, devaluation of the therapist and therapy, and seemingly contradictory risk-taking behaviors which jeopardize their stated goals.

In addition, consequences of the brain injury often include an altered capacity for insight, a reduced ability to identify the sources of one's own distress, or difficulty in recognizing, understanding, or anticipating the consequences of one's own behavior. Thus, in order to be effective, counseling must not only facilitate a person's capacity for self-determination in the face of external barriers, but also help clients gain access to and awareness of the inner psychological processes which influence their decisions. In this regard, counseling and psychotherapy with a client having a traumatic brain injury is no different from any other. It does require, however, that the counselor understand the various ways in which the traumatic brain injury may be manifested and the common cognitive, emotional, and personality disturbances which can occur.

Psychological disturbances after traumatic brain injury

The discussion of psychological disturbances after traumatic brain injury will include changes in thinking, feeling, or behaving that influence the person's ability to function as well as his self-image and self-esteem. Prigatano (1996)[2] and others have suggested that psychological disturbances after brain injury can be classified according to three categories. The first consists of neuropsychologically mediated problems which arise as a direct consequence of organic damage. The second category consists of emotionally based problems that are related to a reaction to the injury or attempts to cope with the effects of the injury. The third category consists of pre-injury personality characteristics which may persist after injury, and influence both the expression of neurologic damage and the person's reactions to injury.

Neuropsychologically mediated and organic problems

In general, there appears to be a fairly consistent association between neurologically based personality and behavioral symptoms and the severity of injury. These symptoms may be especially prominent during the early stage of recovery and coincide with the period of cognitive disorganization. For example, it is not uncommon for hospitalized clients to become extremely agitated and even combative once they have begun emerging from coma. This probably represents a period in which a person is more responsive to various sources of stimulation in his or her environment, yet still lacks the cognitive ability to either filter out irrelevant stimulation or make complete sense of their surroundings. The agitation may be accompanied by gross misunderstandings or distortions of what is going on around them, as well as apparently bizarre interpretations in an attempt to make sense of their environment. At this stage, it is not unusual for the person to misidentify the hospital as a hotel, or to believe that they are at work. This may coincide with a period of post-traumatic amnesia, in which the person's ability to recall information from moment to moment is dramatically reduced, so that older and more familiar memories are more easily recalled and will intrude on current events. Thus, it is the combination of direct changes in the functioning of nervous tissue and the accompanying cognitive limitations that underlies this type of psychological disturbance. It can be important to recognize these behaviors as neuropsychologically based confabulations or misperceptions rather than as any form of psychiatric disturbance.

This same combination of neurologic and cognitive components can be seen with more persisting behavioral abnormalities. For example, clients may have difficulty controlling their temper or experience periodic angry outbursts. Frequently, there will appear to be minimal or no provocation for these episodes. Yet they probably represent, once again, a *reduced tolerance* for levels of stimulation which had previously been tolerated, along with the *disinhibition* and the full release of an accompanying emotional response. Even in cases of relatively mild traumatic brain injury, an increase in irritability and loss of patience are among the personality changes most commonly reported by clients and (especially) by family members.

In many cases, the degree of psychological and behavioral disturbance appears to be related to the overall degree of injury and the extent of neurologic damage. This may be particularly with head trauma, in which the diffuse disruption of nerve fibers extending throughout the brain is one of the primary mechanisms of injury. There are also behavioral abnormalities, however, which may be related to particularly focal areas of injury. In traumatic brain injury, both the frontal and the anterior temporal lobes are particularly susceptible to confusion due to the bony structures of the skull in these areas. Both the frontal and temporal lobes are known to regulate various types of socially appropriate behaviors and emotional reactions, so that damage to one or both of these areas may again increase the potential for neurologically mediated behavior problems or personality chances.

Pepping and Roueche (1990)[3] have summarized many of the personality and cognitive changes which may result from neurologic damage. Among the personality changes considered to be organically based are the following:

1. Egocentricity and loss of ability to show empathy (frontal)
2. Poor social judgment, impulsive or inappropriate social behavior (frontal)
3. Disinhibition of emotional reactions, thoughts, or actions (frontal)
4. Loss of the self-critical attitude (frontal)
5. Childish or silly behaviors, euphoria (frontal)
6. Apathy, lack of concern, and lack of motivation
7. Emotional liability, mood swings, inappropriate laughing or crying (frontal, temporal, frontotemporal)
8. Increased irritability and aggression (temporal)
9. Suspiciousness, paranoia, misperception of the intention of others (temporal, parietal)
10. Catastrophic reactions (frontal, temporal, diffuse)

When considering possible neuropsychologically mediated behavior problems, it is also important to recognize the contribution of cognitive deficits. Among the most common deficits after traumatic brain injury are reduced attention and concentration and heightened distractibility. This may result in difficulty following instructions or learning new information; probably more importantly, the client may look as if he is not paying attention despite repeated requests to do so. Attentional deficits are likely to be most prominent when the client is required to pay attention to more than one thing at a time. This may prove impossible to do, although the client is capable of performing each activity one at a time.

Memory problems are also particularly prominent, and are among the symptoms most likely to be identified by clients and their families as presenting problems. Reduced learning ability and poor memory are among the principal problems associated with poor work performance, as will be discussed more fully below. Not only may they interfere with the acquisition of job skills, but they may also result in poor work behaviors. We have been notified of clients who failed to return from a lunch break because they forgot that they were at work!

Difficulty with executive functioning such as reduced initiation and persistence on a task, poor planning ability, reduced organization, and difficulty correcting errors are frequently a consequence of traumatic brain injury. These deficits will obviously interfere with a person's ability to function without supervision. It is not uncommon to see dissociation between a client's intact ability to *verbally describe* a procedure or appropriate social response and his impaired ability to *actually perform* the required response. In many cases, his inability to perform is related to defects in speed of information processing. Not surprisingly, this can create the impression that the client is simply unwilling to respond appropriately or that they are noncompliant.

Emotional reactions to injury

Emotional reactions after injury appear to be particularly related to the recognition of reduced competencies, and more generally, a sense of loss of self. Unlike the neurologically mediated problems, emotional reactions appear to bear no consistent relationship to the neurologic severity of injury. In addition, the degree of emotional distress and difficulty adjusting to the effects of the injury frequently increase over time.

During the acute period, there may be little evidence that clients are experiencing any emotional distress although their behavior is inappropriate and disorganized; in fact, there may be little awareness of difficulty. As the client experiences repeated or prolonged difficulty, or as it becomes apparent that the extent of recovery of work or social functioning is not going to be as great as expected or hoped for, emotional reactions may worsen.

Depression is a common reaction to the losses sustained by a person with a traumatic brain injury. Increases in cognitive ability and self-awareness over time may be accompanied by increased recognition of deficits, and increasing depression. The attempt to return to work may be the first time that the client really confronts the discrepancies between his or her current level of functioning and pre-injury abilities. It is not uncommon to see a period of elation on returning to work, followed by increasing sadness and disappointment. The most significant symptoms of a clinical depression are subjective feelings of sadness and depressed mood, and the loss of interest or pleasure in usual activities. Additional symptoms include poor appetite or overeating, sleep disturbance, fatigue or lack of energy, low self-esteem, feelings of worthlessness, excessive guilt, and difficulty concentrating or making decisions. Depression, as an accompaniment to increased self-awareness, may be reconceptualized even to the client as a step in getting better or adjusting. Anxiety, while probably less prominent than depression, may be particularly evident in clients attempting to avoid detection of their deficits or embarrassment. There may be an avoidance of the work setting, or other people in the work setting. Feelings of mistrust, isolation, and social withdrawal may become prominent if the anxiety persists. Medications are sometimes helpful during the adjustment period, particularly with aggression.

In general, fluctuations in a client's emotional reactions to injury are not uncommon as they experience varying degrees of adjustment and awareness. These changes are also accompanied by, and influenced by changes in the level of acceptance, understanding, and tolerance exhibited by family, friends, employers, and others.

Pre-injury personality characteristics

Pre-injury personality characteristics may be exaggerated after injury; other clients may show drastic alterations or reversals of their personality traits. it is important to obtain information and an adequate understanding of a person's premorbid functioning before attributing changes in behavior to the effects of the injury. We have frequently started to treat patients for varying behavioral abnormalities only to discover with further exploration that this was probably not very different from their pre-injury functioning. The client's coping style and responses to stressful situations before the injury need to be explored. Tendencies toward minimization or amplification of emotional situations, adaptability to change, willingness to consider psychological explanations for one's behavior, and tolerance for interpersonal disclosure are all likely to be carried over and influence the person's response to injury and to treatment.

Similarly, family relationships, including the need for affiliation and level of dependency within the family system will influence treatment. We have found it helpful to examine at least two dimensions of family functioning. First, the degree to which the family system considers itself responsible (or at fault) for the client's disability. Second, the degree to which the family system holds itself accountable for the client's future.

Social functioning and status need to be considered. Various forms of risk-taking and sensation-seeking, as well as substance use or abuse, may be common among the persons at greatest risk to sustain a traumatic brain injury.

In general, pre-existing personality, coping, family, and socialization factors probably represent respective limitations, although not necessarily contra-indications, to therapy.

Psychological assessment

An important responsibility of the counselor working with clients who have traumatic brain injury is the recognition and differentiation among these various psychological disturbances. Obviously, differing combinations of organic, emotional, and characterological disorders may exist, and at times it may not be possible to isolate any single component. However, familiarity with the various possible presentations will increase the likelihood of an appropriate therapeutic intervention. For example, a 35-year-old man was referred for a psychological evaluation by his rehabilitation counselor, specifically for assessment of depression and possible malingering. The client had sustained a closed head injury two and one-half years earlier, and although he had been severely injured, he had made good neurologic recovery and been discharged from the hospital after two months with no apparent deficits. He then returned to his job as a loan officer, but was unable to follow through with any previous accounts and was temporarily assigned to assist another bank officer. However, he continued to repeatedly enter his old office, manipulate his old accounts, and generally behave as if he had never been absent from his job, despite being told several times not to do so. Shortly after, he was given a medical leave of absence and recommended for a psychiatric evaluation. He did see a psychiatrist (although he did not understand the reason for the referral, he complied in order to not lose his job) who diagnosed a depression with psychomotor retardation and placed him on anti-depressant medication. He had been unable to return to work since that time. Although he attempted to do so on several occasions, he would become disruptive and verbally insulting to his supervisors, and he was then eventually released.

On the psychological evaluation, he stated that he would still like to return to his former job, and still thought he would be able to do so with no difficulty. With direct questioning he admitted to having some memory problems which might limit his ability to perform his former work, but when asked to name three other jobs he would like to do he could only suggest becoming a supervisor at his former bank. When questioned about the impact of his injury on his daily functioning, he again acknowledged some forgetfulness, with an apparent lack of concern. He spent his time watching television and did little else around the house, neglecting home maintenance activities and his former hobby as a locksmith. When questioned about this, he stated that he still enjoyed his hobby, but all his equipment was downstairs in the basement and although he was physically able to walk downstairs he preferred not to. His wife reported that he used to be very outgoing, but now rarely interacted with family or friends. He had become much more compliant in acquiescing to her suggestions or preferences, and he was less motivated and rarely initiated or followed through on any action on his own. Although usually withdrawn since the injury, he had made several verbal outbursts lasting several minutes, after which he was either very remorseful or denied that the incident had even occurred. He had little understanding of why he had been let go from his work, did not recall any inappropriate behaviors or conflicts with his supervisors, and, in general, saw no reason why he could not return to work at any time.

While this man exhibited no depressed mood or loss of interests, he certainly had a reduced awareness of his deficits and an inability to recognize the impact of his social behaviors, as well as a general reduction in activity level and initiation. He had never appreciated that he was unable to perform his prior job, and in his mind had been subjected to repeated, senseless changes and frustrations. With a program of education regarding his neurologic injury and neuropsychological deficits, counseling to assist him identify aspects of his behavior which were different from his prior self (including the effect of his memory deficits on work and daily functioning), and perhaps most importantly a structured, consistent system of behavioral supervision (both at home and at the bank) he was able to return to employment. It still remained necessary for him to work at a much reduced capacity. While intervention did not, certainly, alleviate this man's neurologic and cognitive disability, he was able to improve his daily functioning, once his behaviors were understood in terms of a neurologically mediated disturbance, rather than either an emotional or volitional disorder.

Counseling interactions and the therapeutic relationship

Basic interaction considerations

While neuropsychologically mediated deficits exhibit a fairly consistent though modest relationship to clients' everyday functioning and employment capabilities, personality and emotional factors exert a significant influence, at least on clients' subjective disability. Chelune, Heaton and Lehman (1986)[4] found that clients' complaints of cognitive, memory, communication and sensorimotor impairments were more strongly related to the results from the Minnesota Multiphasic Personality inventory than to their neuropsychological test performance. In particular, the clients' levels of emotional distress discriminated between those who minimized their disability, irrespective of actual neuropsychological impairment based on test results. Changes in levels of emotional distress over the course of brain injury rehabilitation appear to vary according to clients' subjective reports of disability and can be related to rehabilitation outcomes (employment status), independent of changes in neuropsychological impairment.[5] On the basis of these studies, it is likely that clients' emotional and personality status will influence their ability to function in everyday life and their ability to return to successful employment, whatever the clients' work skills and level of ability may be. These factors, therefore, need to be considered within the context of any counseling or therapeutic approach.

In addition to the potential impact of cognitive deficits on daily living and vocational functioning, these impairments will influence the nature and success of therapeutic interactions. Given the emphasis on verbal interaction and self-observation characteristic of many counseling therapies, deficits in language and self-awareness require specific consideration. Clients frequently will have difficulty with complex language, with abstract language, and with the use of metaphor. This is not limited to clients who are frankly (or even subtly) aphasic, but may be secondary to problems attending to lengthy or complex conversation, remembering difficult or abstract prose material, or with higher-level reasoning. Basic considerations for the counselor include the reliance on simple sentence structure, the avoidance of overly long statements, the use of specific examples, and remaining sensitive to the client's level of understanding. Fordyce (1999)[6] suggests covering a limited finite set of issues per session — the topics to be covered should be prioritized and organized, which becomes increasingly important with the client who has more severe neuropsychological impairment. It is not effective to rely on a client's facial expression or body language or gauge his understanding, since this may not be accurate. Confused by unnecessary, complex, abstract, or metaphorical language, the client may add to the confusion by giving nonverbal or verbal indicators that he understands the content of the language when in fact he is totally missing the boat. All too frequently, clients exhibit an altogether concrete interpretation of metaphorical language ("well, if you miss the boat, you might not get out of here, or you could be late coming home") or an inability to extract meaning from complex language (e.g., compound sentences, sentences which convey more than one meaning, or sentences which carry many pieces of information). It is useful to have the client paraphrase the therapist's statements at different points in the interaction to insure that he understands the meaning and the intent of the communication. It can be particularly important for the client to paraphrase and/or write down therapy directions or homework at a session's end.

Fordyce (1999)[6] suggests that repetition in these counseling sessions is often a positive. If clients have difficulty with a receptive or expressive language difficulty or aphasia, they need encouragement to let the therapist know. Pragmatic means of communication may need to be developed — sometimes using pictures, charts or graphs.

Clients with reduced self-awareness may not understand the nature of the counseling relationship, and may be likely to misinterpret the therapist's intentions. Clients may be unable to understand the meaning of the therapist's interventions or to relate these interventions to their own situation. There may be little appreciation for the way in which their deficits affect their functioning, and so they may not see the reason for being in treatment. This may be mistaken for a lack of concern or motivation, when in fact it would be more accurately considered a lack of awareness. Development of the capacity for self-observation may itself be a primary goal of psychotherapy after traumatic brain injury.[7]

The therapist is advised to develop a method for interrupting and redirecting clients with impaired self-awareness in order to avoid tangential discussion or hyperverbosity.[6] Politely listening to tangent conversation is often not very assistive to the client (e.g., hand signals to increase focus can even be effective when previously discussed with the client). Fordyce (1999)[6] suggests balancing bad news with client strengths — as opposed to emphasizing — deficits underscore the benefits of realizing and dealing with impairment. Every effort should be made to modulate stresses for the client with anger management issues (using a non-threatening posture, supportive time outs, etc.), as necessary.

Uomoto (1997)[8] states that pragmatically, given a significant level of altered awareness, the therapist may have to assist the client in drawing conclusions and then guide the client through the behavioral rationales and themes that lead to the conclusions. He also emphasizes the use of a therapy log, not only to record conclusions, insights, observations, etc., but also to record homeworks. These logs can be reviewed at the beginning of each new session. The structure of the therapy session might also be altered depending upon the benefit to the client. The length of the session might be shortened (e.g., to 30-45 minutes) and significant others brought in to specific sessions to improve generalization strategies (e.g., anger management) to the home.

In general, therapeutic interactions should not rely solely on verbal or even pictorial interventions. For example, modeling of behaviors by the therapist and rehearsal of behaviors by the client can usually be incorporated into the therapy interaction without difficulty. These behavioral interventions help to monitor clients' comprehension and ability to take messages outside of the therapy room.

The role of the therapeutic alliance has been recognized as a crucial key to change in diverse forms of therapy, but has been given remarkably little attention in the rehabilitation of clients with traumatic brain injury. The therapeutic alliance has three basic characteristics: client-therapist expectancies and belief in the helping relationship, client-therapist collaboration on the goals and tasks of therapy, and client commitment especially as gauged through defensiveness and resistance to treatment.

Client—therapist expectancies

The establishment of a common expectation and the initial conceptualization of treatment are essential aspects of the counseling process. One of the most important functions of the counseling relationship is to provide clients with a framework to explore the notions of illness and health, normality and disability. The treatment should provide clients with a rationale for their "illness behavior" and enable them to make sense of their symptoms. The initial phases of counseling may be largely didactic, dealing with issues of structural damage to the brain and permanent loss of function, and providing realistic estimates of a clients' future, without precluding the possibility of change and taking away hope and motivation. The therapist may need to address issues of not only "what has happened to me?" but also "why has this happened to me?"[2]

Clients and therapists alike bring with them into the relationship various attributions regarding past performance and treatment possibilities. Clients may tend to underestimate their deficits[5] while clinicians may tend to overdiagnose pathology.[9]

The rehabilitation process may generate additional attributions regarding patient change. We have periodically surveyed clients and therapists involved in a brain injury rehabilitation program regarding their beliefs about the reasons for patient improvement, or lack of improvement, in therapy.[10] Both rehabilitation clients and therapists appear to identify client variables, that is, clients' cognitive, emotional and physical deficits as the primary obstacles to their resuming pre-injury level of functioning. However, among these types of deficits, differences emerge between clients' and therapists' views. Clients are much more likely to attribute their problems to residual physical deficits, and generally minimize the impact of their cognitive deficits. This appears to be a rather robust belief. Clients expressed this opinion whether they were rating themselves, other clients with whom they were familiar, or a prototypical client with a head injury. In addition, there was no relationship between clients' own level of neuropsychological impairment and their tendency to attribute importance to physical rather than cognitive factors. (Emotional factors were considered slightly more important than cognitive factors; this appeared to be particularly true for clients who were further post-injury.) Therapists, on the other hand, gave much greater emphasis to the clients' residual cognitive deficits as reasons for their disability, while generally minimizing their physical deficits. This was true for all disciplines. (Interestingly, emotional factors were this time considered slightly more important than physical factors, and less important than the clients themselves rated them.)

Among therapy variables, the differences in attributions of success and failure are perhaps more striking. Therapists appear to attribute client's improvement to the therapy, while they attribute lack of progress to the clients' lack of motivation or maintaining unrealistic expectations. Clients are more likely to attribute gains to their own motivation, as well as to the support of family members. They cite the lack of appropriate therapy, not receiving enough therapy, and inadequacy of social support systems as reasons for their lack of improvement. In general, it appears that both clients and therapists attribute success to things over which they have control and they attribute failure to factors beyond their control.

It is likely that these client-therapist expectancies exert significant influence over the therapeutic process, and may in themselves be important determinants of success and failure. It, therefore, appears to be important to align client-therapist expectancies throughout treatment. This process should begin during the initial interview with the client, in order to determine what the client expects from treatment and to clarify what the therapist believes himself or herself is to provide. The client should also be encouraged to be open about any preconceptions of the process of therapy, and these issues can be acknowledged and addressed directly. At the same time, possible resistances to the treatment can begin to be anticipated.

Various procedures can be utilized to better engage and prepare the client for therapy. Those procedures that attempt to alter the client's expectations to match the therapy are referred to as *role induction* procedures.[11] In general, role induction procedures include efforts to prepare the client for therapy and include three types of interventions: instructional methods, observational and participatory learning, and treatment contracting.

Instructional methods of role induction include written and verbal information about the nature of therapy or the counseling interaction and descriptions of various behaviors which might be expected from the client. These might include the number and frequency of sessions; the length and type of service; the conditions leading to discharge; the nature and frequency of homework assignments; the types of behaviors which the therapist may address (e.g., emotional symptoms, social skills, unrealistic expectations) and the types of behaviors expected from the client (e.g., self-disclosure, consideration of alternative choices, unpaid volunteer work). This type of intervention appears to be especially suited for clients for whom an initial resistance to treatment might be expected to compromise their full understanding of and participation in the counseling process.

Observational and participatory learning procedures allow the client to practice the role in therapy but outside of the actual treatment. One form of this might be to have clients observe a group session without being required to participate, or to provide the client with the opportunity to talk to another client about their experience in therapy. This is not that different from the use of group therapy to allow clients the chance to share their experiences and overcome their sense of isolation through group involvement, except that it is used as a means of preparing the client for treatment. Another participatory learning procedure is to provide the client with the opportunity to meet with someone other than the counselor every three or four sessions, to discuss relationship problems that may arise during therapy. The goal of this intervention is to provide clients with information, suggestions, and reinforcement which can enable them to address the problems within their therapy session. This procedure can assist in maintaining their engagement in counseling. The use of observational and participatory learning procedures may be of particular value for clients with significant cognitive impairments. In some cases, this will allow the counselor to provide services to clients who would otherwise be unable to participate in counseling. Since therapy engagement would generally be unlikely for many individuals with pre-existing personality disorders, approaches such as these may also help to attract or retain these types of clients in therapy.

Therapeutic contracting has been widely used in counseling and psychotherapy and is typically successful in attempting to maintain compliance and reduce client drop out. When used in this manner, the goal is to provide the client with a framework that enables him to make explicit the expectations for treatment, rather than prescribing specific forms of behavior change. Most often, this will involve the establishment of a specific treatment goal or a time-limited course of therapy. The use of time-limited therapy contracting often increases the probability that clients will complete their course of treatment. A serendipitous finding from time-limited therapy is that on average these clients remain in treatment for longer periods of time than do clients in open-ended therapy.[11] Therapeutic contracting should typically include the following components:

1. The time limits of treatment should be specified. This limit may include a provision for extension or renewal based upon the review of the effectiveness of treatment.
2. The goals of treatment to be accomplished during the time period should be specified, even when it is expected that these may change over the course of the treatment.
3. The contract should represent the expected roles and behaviors of the therapist as well as the expected roles of the client.

4. The consequences of failing to comply with the contract should be specified.
5. The treatment contract may be written out and signed by both parties, in order to maintain a focus on the conditions of treatment and refer back to as necessary.

In using therapeutic contracts with clients with brain injuries, we have found it to be particularly useful in those cases where the complexity of the client's situation or the tendency of the client to incorporate multiple foci into treatment threatens to forestall any appreciable progress. For example, one 28-year-old woman had sustained a severe traumatic brain injury 11 years earlier, and continued to have significant physical and behavioral limitations as well as frequent seizures which prevented her from working consistently or living alone. The seizures required continual medical supervision, but they continued and were a source of social embarrassment to her. She had not been allowed to leave home and live on her own as would have been age-appropriate behavior, which increased her sense of dependency and resentment towards her parents. This had led to multiple episodes of running away, alcohol abuse and sexual promiscuity, and two prior suicide attempts. She had received several courses of cognitive and vocational rehabilitation and had several supported employment placements. She had initially done well on each of these until an episode of seizures or behavioral dyscontrol occurred. As various issues were addressed in treatment, the client appeared to shift the focus of her complaints to another area. This not only prevented therapy from adequately addressing her various problems, but also reinforced the view that her situation was hopeless. Contracting in this case was effective in negotiating priorities with her, establishing a hierarchical treatment plan and timetable, and in getting this client to agree to see each problem through to some form of resolution.

We have also found the therapeutic contract to be useful when working with clients who have relatively mild residual deficits, and who have already been through at least one course of appropriate therapy, yet who seek to make further change. In these cases, the use of a time-limited contract serves several functions: it allows the opportunity to promote further gains when the chance of doing so is really rather limited; it makes explicit the expectation that substantial change is unlikely; it removes the onus of failure from both client and therapist if, in fact, change does not occur; and it allows the therapist to reframe the client's expectation, i.e., "Now I can assure myself that I've made every effort to improve to my maximum potential, and I'm ready to move on as I am." A therapeutic contract may also be applied within an individual treatment session, to maintain a focus on a specific goal within that session.

While we have referred to these procedures as methods to alter clients' expectancies, in reality they are also methods which require therapists to adjust expectations and adapt the treatment process to meet clients' needs and abilities to utilize therapy. The essence of the client-therapist relationship is the client's belief in the therapist's ability and desire to help.

Dunbar (1980)[12] has noted that therapist behaviors such as "hurriedness, interruptions, lack of time for listening, inattentiveness, and not identifying the patient's problems from the patient's own perspective, will interfere with the therapist's approachability" (p. 80) and limit the therapist's effectiveness. In working with a client with a brain injury who may have specific issues related to the injury, disability, and treatment, the therapist needs to demonstrate his or her understanding and acceptance of the client. One should be able to discuss with clients the neurologic, cognitive, and social aspects of their condition. The therapist needs to understand the traumatic nature of the injury, and the sudden and irreversible disjunction of the present condition from the pre-injury situation.

Clients with brain injury need to be accepted for who they are as well as for who they may become. Because of their cognitive limitations, interventions may need to be repeated regularly and may seem to be delivered without any effect. This can tempt the therapist to underestimate or even abandon the relationship. We have been frequently impressed, however, by the emotional impact the relationship has carried in the absence of overt acknowledgments by the client. In fact, the establishment and maintenance of an interpersonal relationship despite the client's physical, cognitive, and social limitations is of tremendous importance to the client with a brain injury.

Client–therapist collaboration

The formation of an effective client–therapist collaboration relies on the therapist's ability to create a shared understanding and conceptualization of therapy, and to negotiate common goals and treatment objectives. In a general rehabilitation setting, the practice of patient and therapist sharing decisions about treatment was more important than interpersonal or affective dimensions of the therapy relationship for the achievement of rehabilitation goals.[13] In a large vocational rehabilitation agency which served a wide variety of patients with neuropsychiatric disabilities, Galano (1977)[14] compared clients for whom no explicit treatment goals were developed, clients who had specific treatment goals determined by their therapist, and clients who actively collaborated with their therapists on the development of their treatment goals. Only active collaboration between therapist and clients on treatment goals resulted in an improvement in the number of treatment goals met or surpassed, and this improvement was not due to differences in the quality or difficulty of the goals established.

In working with clients after brain injury, the ability to form an active-collaborative relationship appears to depend on several client characteristics. These include the organic bases of awareness, severity of cognitive impairments and cognitive disorganization, motivation and behavioral capacity to actively participate in therapy, level of psychological distress, and defensiveness and need to exert control. There are various actions that the therapist can take to address these issues and facilitate the collaborative relationship.

Difficulties in awareness that result from neurologic injury may be persistent and limit the client's ability to apply compensations or participate in therapy.[15] Crosson et al.[15] have described three types and levels of awareness deficits which may result from brain injury. *Intellectual awareness* is the ability to understand at some level that a particular disability exists. At the simplest level, the client may recognize or acknowledge that something is difficult for them. At another level, the client may be able to identify a number of activities which are difficult and recognize the similarities among them. A higher level of intellectual awareness "is required to recognize the implications of one's deficits, for example, that visuospatial deficits might hamper a career in graphic design."[15]

Clients who are able to describe their deficits, yet fail to see the implications of these same impairments for returning to work, may be particularly frustrating. They can appear to be stubborn or uncooperative in therapy. It is, therefore, important to understand that this may represent different levels of intellectual awareness.

Intellectual awareness serves as the basis for two further types of awareness. *Emergent awareness* is the ability of a client to recognize a problem while it is actually occurring. *Anticipatory awareness* is the ability to foresee that a problem is likely to occur under certain circumstances because of a deficit. Once again, the therapist needs to understand the possible independence between lower and high levels of awareness. For example, the bank loan officer could eventually describe how his memory deficits and calculation difficulties would prevent him from making certain necessary computations (thus showing intellectual awareness), yet he repeatedly attempted to open new files requiring these very computations whenever he returned to his work (an emergent awareness deficit). *Organic awareness* deficits are probably related to various cognitive impairments.

Cognitive impairments may also limit the client's ability to anticipate treatment goals and directions or to understand the relationship between the treatment content and the client's own desires. Goal setting should, therefore, be specific, tangible and concrete. Several guidelines for setting treatment goals are appropriate for these clients:

1. *Establish a well-defined treatment focus:* Many clients with head injury and certainly those who exhibit any significant degree of cognitive disorganization will have difficulty appreciating vague or abstract treatment objectives. Treatment goals should be clearly specified and tied to specific behaviors expected from the client. Thus, it is almost always preferable to maintain a focus on specific, behavioral target symptoms rather than complex interpersonal or personality dynamics. Clients may also benefit from being given a choice from a limited number of treatment goals, rather than leaving it open-ended. This

enlists them in the process of making relevant treatment decisions while reducing the level of cognitive complexity.

2. *Set proximal goals.* It is easier to maintain focus on a goal that the client can attain within a reasonable amount of time, and receive direct concrete feedback. For example, setting a goal of completing four out of five math problems correctly this week may be more effective in maintaining the client's involvement and participation than the goal of balancing the checkbook for the month or completing a math course.

3. *Use mediating goals.* The relationship between the proximal goals and the eventual functional ability should be made explicit. These can be conceptualized as the steps required to move the client from his current status to achievement of a desired outcome.

4. *Use comprehensive checks.* The client's understanding of the reason for a given activity or intervention should be monitored by having the client repeat or paraphrase this information. This should be done at least every session or every time a new goal or activity is established. Written information can be provided, or graphic charts and time frames can be utilized to provide the client with a frame of reference and sense of progress.

5. *Teach goal setting:* The skill of setting goals can be incorporated into therapy as a structured, formal activity similar to that used for problem solving. A simple procedure involves having the client define the initial state ("This is my situation now") and goal state ("This is what I want to be doing") and decide on a series of steps that will lead from one to the other.

Cognitive deficits can also affect the client's access to internal verbalizations which mediate much behavior and reduce his capability to perform accurate appraisals of his emotional state and its source. It is frequently difficult for clients with head injuries to get over emotions once they have been aroused, resulting in prolonged discomfort. This inability to moderate levels of emotional arousal or to attribute feelings to real situational stressors may limit the client's ability to participate in treatment. Pine (1985)[16] has described several techniques for use with the fragile patient, which can be applied to working with clients with brain injuries:

1. *Limit the client's responses to a situation or statement made by the therapist.* It may be useful to provide a label to the client's expression of affect, and to attempt to relate the feeling to a specific source or reason (e.g., "You seem to be getting angry now. I can understand if you feel angry when we talk about your old job.").

2. *Postpone dealing with difficult issues until the client's emotional state has subsided or at points in the session when he is able to better control his emotional response.* ("Earlier we were speaking about your old jobs. I

want to understand why that makes you angry. Let's talk about that
now.")
3. *Maximize the client's preparedness and the supportive aspects of the environment.* For example, the therapist might state "I want to talk about
something which may make you feel angry...listen to what I say and
then we can talk about it...alright?"

An apparent lack of motivation to engage in therapy can result from
clients' lack of understanding about the goals of therapy or lack of understanding or acknowledgement of their own symptoms. Neurobehavioral
problems, such as reduced initiation, poor follow-through, and difficulty
formulating future-oriented goals can limit a client's capacity to be an active
participant in treatment. The client's participation can be enlisted initially
by using the procedures discussed above to establish agreement between
client and therapist expectations. Beyond that, the therapist may adapt an
attitude of active questioning, encouraging and cajoling the client to contribute his own observations, and soliciting the client's suggestions as to how
to proceed with treatment. The client might be encouraged to explore the
validity of symptoms or deficits, and particularly to search for similarities
among situations where he has or might experience difficulty, with the
therapist using what Meichenbaum (1985)[17] refers to as the *Columbo routine
of befuddlement* to increase a client's activity and responsibilty within treatment. The client can also be encouraged to disagree with the therapist, to
disprove the validity of the therapist's observtions, and to generate his own
alternative treatment goals and directions. These procedures may temporarily increase a client's feelings of discomfort with therapy, and care needs
to be taken to provide appropriate support.

Active collaboration can sometimes be achieved by incorporating some
or all of the above suggestions into a procedure of *prescriptive self-monitoring,*
which involves clients being asked to make specific observations and records
of daily functioning outside of the treatment setting, to develop appropriate
treatment goals. The form of self-monitoring may range from open-ended
notes or a diary to specific checklists, and observations may vary from
external signs of other people's reactions to the client's personal inner
thoughts and feelings. Use of prescriptive self-monitoring can follow several
basic principles to promote the client's participation:

1. *The client should be allowed to suggest the specific behaviors to be monitored.*
   In fact, the client may suggest the self-monitoring procedure itself;
   the therapist may merely express puzzlement over how to go about
   understanding what the client is all about, or confusion at the lack of
   behaviors appropriate for therapy, and ask the client for suggestions
   as to how the therapist can learn more about the client.
2. *The self-monitoring procedure should be kept simple.* The client will have
   more success monitoring one or two simple behaviors than keeping
   track of multiple symptoms or contingencies. Less frequent intervals

of monitoring (e.g., morning and evening) may be easier than hourly intervals or recordings of every occurrence.

3. *Self-monitoring of difficulties can be uncomfortable, and many clients will express some discomfort over having to note their difficulties, either because of the emotional consequences or the awkwardness of self-observation and recording.* This discomfort and difficulty should be appreciated by the therapist. It is sometimes helpful to anticipate with the client the possible discomforts as well as the difficulties in keeping up the self-monitoring procedure, while encouraging the client to persist with his worthwhile endeavor.

4. *Reinforce the fact that it is the client's idea that prescriptive self-monitoring be conducted, or at least that he has agreed to do so.* It is also good to reinforce how helpful the information will be to the therapist and therapeutic process (e.g., "So, what you've come up with is a way to keep track of those times when you might get in trouble by not paying attention. You think this probably happens more with your wife than your boss, but we're not sure about that. This is great, and will really help me understand what's happening with you during the week.").

5. *Use the information obtained from self-monitoring, whatever the results.* Even when clients have been unable to unwilling to maintain the self-monitoring outside of sessions, or when they have not observed any difficulties, this information can be incorporated into the treatment session and developed into a treatment focus. The value of prescriptive self-monitoring lies in the facilitation of the active-collaborative role on the part of the client.

For the client who remains unable to become actively engaged in treatment, this lack of collaboration needs to be confronted within the treatment session. One of the most common errors of treatment is the failure to approach the client who presents as uninvolved in treatment. Although confrontation sometimes acquires a negative connotation in rehabilitation, it remains an effective therapist intervention which need not be hostile or threatening. Interventions — to create a situation where the client *experiences* a discrepancy between the expected and actual level of performance, or between a therapist's and client's views of treatment may be effective in enlisting the client's active participation in the treatment process. In our opinion, there is little risk in the use of confrontation in therapy if the preliminary stages of establishing a shared set of expectancies and a belief in the benevolent intentions of the therapist have been achieved. The failure to establish the client as an active participant is more detrimental to therapy than the possible negative consequences of confrontation conducted within the therapeutic relationship.

Client commitment, denial, and resistance

The subjective lack of appreciation for the existence or severity of deficits after injury represents a particular area of significance for clients with head injury and will often greatly influence the client's commitment to therapy. The issue of denial is, therefore, of central concern to the rehabilitation counseling process. Although denial of illness has been identified as a consequence of a variety of diseases,[18] the particular concerns regarding the client with a traumatic brain injury appear predicated on the assumption that the denial process interferes with the processes of rehabilitation, psychosocial adaptation, and vocational adjustment. The patient referred for counseling who promptly denies having any problems, represents a particular source of challenge, and potential frustration, for the therapist attempting to deliver treatment. Not surprisingly, these clients may have limited ability to utilize, or benefit from, treatment. Should these clients continue to deny or minimize any problems, despite the therapist's best efforts, they may be considered to be resisting treatment. Furthermore, clients who fail to acknowledge their real limitations may assume excessive vocational or social responsibilities, fail to recognize or compensate for their errors, and have difficulty accepting assistance.

Rehabilitation professionals typically assume that awareness and acknowledgment of deficits are associated with more effective treatment and better outcomes. Prigatano (1986)[2] and others indicated that patients with better rehabilitation outcomes exhibited better emotional and motivational functioning, based on relatives' reports. Fordyce and Roueche (1986)[5] identified two groups of patients based upon patient, family, and staff ratings of competency prior to treatment. One group rated themselves similar to the ratings of staff, whereas the other group exhibited a pronounced tendency to underestimate their level of impairment when compared with staff members' estimations. The latter group was further subdivided on the basis of change in patients' ratings relative to staff ratings over the course of rehabilitation. In one group, patient and staff ratings became more similar, whereas for the other group, the differences in perspective and beliefs about level of impairment actually increased. Among the patients who showed increased awareness of deficits, 78% were engaged in productive activity following their rehabilitation; but among the patients with persistent lack of awareness of deficits, only 25% were engaged in productive activity.

Clinically, these findings suggest that for clients unable to make a commitment to treatment due to their unawareness of deficits, priority needs to be given to addressing the client's awareness deficits and resistance to therapy. A goal of counseling can be to increase the client's capacity for self-observation, which might be accomplished by providing them with specific, objective feedback and emphasizing the educative and informative aspects of therapy.

The use of videotape can be effective in providing clients with feedback about their interpersonal and communication skills.[19] Such feedback can be repeated as required by the client to compensate for attention, memory, or comprehension deficits. In addition, repeated observations of their videotaped performance may allow clients to more objectively evaluate their own behavior. Videotapes of clients' performances can be used to actually teach them and have them practice the skills of self-monitoring and self-assessment. For example, we have frequently used a relatively simple sensorimotor task and had clients evaluate themselves as correct or incorrect after each trial. Despite the relative simplicity of this procedure, many clients have difficulty evaluating their performance accurately. Clients are then shown a tape of another person imitating the movements, and asked to judge whether they were imitated correctly (i.e., the same) or incorrectly (i.e., differently). Next, the clients are shown the tape of them performing the task and asked to judge their own performance from the videotape. Finally, they are given practice in evaluating their own performance in real time.

This same objective self-awareness training procedure can be utilized with tasks and work behaviors of increasing complexity. Formal checklists and behavioral self-monitoring inventories can also be incorporated into a variety of settings and adapted to review the occurrence of any number of functional or interpersonal behaviors. Given the opportunity for structured self-observation, clients' behavior will often show a reactive change in the desired direction, and this therapeutic change can be further enhanced by providing them with feedback about the accuracy of their self-observations.[20] These findings suggest that overt self-observation may compensate for the loss of internalized self-monitoring.

Another intervention for decreased awareness is the use of community–based activities (e.g., work trials and situational assessments) that place the client in real-life activities, and avoid the artificially and arbitrariness of the treatment environment. Clients can have an active role in selecting the setting and activity for such interventions, based on their previous activities or future plans. This approach typically has increased face validity and meaningfulness for many clients and may also provide salient feedback about their real-life performance. Additionally, this treatment approach appears to transfer some of the control of treatment from therapist to client, which can increase compliance and reduce one potential source of emotional distress. Cues from the work environment and from co-workers assist in increasing clients' self-awareness and social awareness, and the therapist can become an ally in the absorption and adaptation processes. The use of community-based and real-life treatment environments appears to be particularly appropriate to vocational issues and can be readily incorporated into place-and-train and job coaching models of vocational rehabilitations.

Individual therapy can also be utilized with the client who exhibits denial or unawareness of deficits. Particular attention can be paid to exploring and defining the client's efficacy expectations (i.e., the client's belief that they will be able to execute specific behaviors leading to desired outcomes).[21] Rather than relying on normative or dichotomous neuropsychological statements about deficits, or the therapist's performance expectancies, the client can be asked to predict his own performance capabilities. This allows the therapist to address the discrepancies between the client's perceived and actual competencies.

Therapeutic interventions can be

1. Verbal and evocative, emphasizing the process of accurate self-appraisal (e.g., "How sure are you that you can do that?" "Are you sure you have done that right? How sure?" "What would it mean if you're unable to do that, but you think you can?");
2. More directive and behaviorally oriented (e.g., "You're still making more mistakes than you said were acceptable. You either have to slow down and correct your own errors...or you could change your goal. Which do you want to do?"); or
3. A combination of both.

The possible relations and implications of the client's deficits to their everyday functioning, including any difficulty in accurately assessing their own performance, can be discussed with them regularly. In offering such interpretations, it is preferable to challenge evidence of the clients' beliefs about their functioning, rather than the beliefs themselves. In general, we agree with Deaton's (1986)[22] suggestion that "all treatments should involve a balance between positive (supportive) and negative (confrontative) elements" (p. 235).

Within the context of a therapeutic alliance, another strategy can be to predict the client's denial. For example, a 24-year-old man with marked impairments in memory and executive function entered post-acute rehabilitation with pronounced denial of any disability and insistence that he could return to work. This denial appeared to represent an inability to integrate the changes in his abilities with his self-concept due to his severe memory deficits, inability to appreciate his limitations in any abstract sense, and the need to avoid becoming emotionally overwhelmed when the deficits were made apparent to him. He rejected any affiliation with other clients, all of whom had "something wrong with their brains" and were, therefore, nothing like him. Instead he fostered a strong association with the various rehabilitation therapists, to whom he referred to as "teachers," who were giving him classes so that he could open his own business. He exhibited a strong identification and personalized relationship with the psychotherapist, whom he regarded as a mentor and potential business partner.

Over the course of treatment, the psychotherapist anticipated for this patient his inevitable frustration with treatment, followed by progressive mistrust and devaluation of his therapists, and his eventual disillusionment with the psychotherapist, as well. A state of unconditional acceptance and support was maintained in psychotherapy despite other difficulties, including his expanding anger and hostility toward the treatment. At the same time, he was encouraged to participate in a process of proximal goal setting, and to identify a concrete and specific progression of steps and mediating goals which would be necessary to enable him to return to his own business. Although not all of the difficulties associated with this client's treatment were avoided, the anticipation of this client's expanding denial and emotional distress increased the therapist's credibility, allowed the client to gradually acknowledge his feelings of dependency and low self-esteem, accept some responsibility for his feelings of anger and his interpersonal problems, and revise his treatment goals without a loss of self-respect. Although, several years later, he continues to exhibit marked reductions in his social and vocational functioning, he has made continued progress in terms of his psychological adjustment and sense of self-worth.

In practice, it is often difficult to differentiate an organic lack of awareness from psychologically and emotionally based denial, or to determine the degree to which they may coexist. In addition, it is likely that the degree of premorbid characterological rigidity and defensiveness is likely to contribute to the person's ability to acknowledge deficits after a head injury. It is, therefore, important to obtain a thorough history and inquire about the client's response to stressful situations, his willingness to acknowledge problems, and to attribute them to psychological or personal causes. (It is worth keeping in mind that most of us tend to attribute difficulties to an external cause; persons who don't are probably being treated for depression.)

Clinical experience suggests that clients who exhibit more extensive and severe neuropsychological deficits often show the least awareness of their disability. This would suggest an organic basis for the decreased awareness. In these cases, it is common for the client to exhibit a reduced awareness of the physical and social environment and diminished interpersonal sensitivity, along with reduced self-monitoring and self-awareness. On the other hand, complaints of disability appear to be related to increased emotional distress and psychopathology, independent of neuropsychological status. This suggests that psychological denial in some cases does represent an emotional reaction and protective response in the face of increasing recognition of disability and distress. Clients may show a normal awareness of the environment, and psychological vigilance in their interpersonal functioning, while offering apparently specific and selective disclaimers regarding their objective deficits. We would propose a simple strategy, which may assist in differentiating between organic and psychological forms of unawareness: If the client is provided with increased information and objective feedback about his deficits, and his ability to acknowledge his deficits increases, then his lack of appreciation for his deficits is probably neurologically mediated. If the client is provided with specific information and evidence regarding his deficit, and there appears to be an increased resistance to acknowledging his limitations and evidence of emotional distress, he is probably exhibiting a protective emotional response.

In some cases, of couse, clients should be allowed to maintain their denial, especially when it does not interfere with therapy or daily functioning. Awareness itself may not be a valuable commodity, and the need for clients to "mourn their deficits" may have more to do with therapists' values and needs than with clients' treatment.[23] Therapists need to consider the client's perspective and respect his experience. In cases where the client continues to be resistant or unable to commit to therapy, he may be resisting an interpretation or treatment plan that is simply untenable or irrelevant to him.

Specific interventions for cognitive and behavioral problems related to vocational rehabilitation procedures and outcomes

It is commonly believed that the cognitive and behavioral problems exhibited by clients with traumatic brain injury are the major obstacles to return to work. Price and Baumann (1990),[1] for example, identified various critical work behaviors considered necessary to succeed in competitive employment. They found that vocationally related difficulties for persons with traumatic brain injury were related to these critical work behaviors rather than to specific job skills and aptitudes. Over 50% of workers with head injuries had problems with work performance, which included behaviors such as exercising good social judgment and presentation. The primary reasons for poor performance in this area were

Acceptance of Worker Role: carrying out work assignments independently (inappropriately), poor judgment in the use of obscenities or playing practical jokes, temperamental behavior.
Degree of Comfort with Supervisor: becoming upset when corrected.
Appropriateness of Personal Relations with Supervisor: discussing personal problems not related to work.
Social Communication Skills: expressing likes and dislikes inappropriately, expressing negative feelings inappropriately, interrupting others while speaking.

The second general dimension related to poor work performance seemed related to cognitive abilities such as learning ability and capacity for self-direction on the job. Over 40% of clients were found to have difficulty in this area of task orientation, which included the following behaviors:

Work Persistence: not maintaining work pace when distractions occurred.
Amount of Supervision Required: inability to recognize their own mistakes, needing more than the average amount of supervision, requiring frequent help with problems.
Work Tolerance: inability to perform tasks that required variety, inability to accept changes in work assignments.

In general, problems with work conformance seemed to be related to social judgment and emotional control, while problems in task orientation were related to cognitive abilities such as sustaining attention, problem solving, mental flexibility, and new learning.

Stapleton, Bennet, and Parenté (1989)[24] obtained reports and behavioral ratings from job coaches who had experience working with clients with traumatic brain injury to determine which behaviors were most problematic on the work site. Major problems were evident in the slow acquisition of job skills, verbal and visual memory, judgment, inflexibility of thinking, and anxiety. Moderate problems on the work site were evident in completion of work in a timely fashion, obsessive/compulsive behavior, inability to detect/correct errors, inability to work independently, attention and concentrations deficits, poor social interaction skills, intellectual limitations, inability to organize/prioritize tasks, difficulty staying on task in the face of distractions, inability to work without structure or make plans independently, and physical limitations.

Once again, most of these problems could be related to two areas. The first included social judgment, planning, insight, and social skills, while the second area included problems in attention and concentration, memory, and new learning. Thus, there appears to be reasonable consistency between these two studies in the identification of the kinds of deficits that are most likely to vocationally impact on clients. These behaviors can serve as a basis for the rehabilitation counselor's interventions. It should be recognized that a client's deficits in these areas, especially at the stage of recovery where the client is attempting vocational re-entry, are likely to be permanent limitations. These interventions are not remedial, but are intended to facilitate the counseling process and perhaps assist the client compensate for residual difficulties.

Interventions and compensations

Learning and acquisition of new job skills.   There is probably a trade-off between speed and accuracy, so that reducing the time spent on new learning may simply increase mistakes. Learning can, however, be facilitated by providing the client with specific instructions and the opportunity to practice new skills. Clients may need to practice new work skills outside of the work environment, which obviously requires more time and effort. The greater the similarity between the training tasks and environment and the actual skills required on the work site, the greater the likelihood that the client will acquire and maintain skills. Overlearning through repetition will typically make the activity more routine and efficient, although such extended training may actually be detrimental if the client is going to be required to perform a variety of different activities.

It is not unusual for clients to require greater amounts of time preparing for their work, to compensate for the greater amount of time required to perform activities while actually on the job. When giving instructions, it is of benefit to obtain a comprehension check from the client by having him repeat or paraphrase the instructions before carrying out the activity. Delays and distractions between the client receiving the instructions and carrying out the activity should be avoided or minimized. (See Chapters six and seven for additional discussion of worker training procedures.)

Error recognition and correction. Clients may be taught to use a formal self-checking routine to detect errors. This will frequently require a step-by-step comparison between the client's actual performance and the job requirements. When an error is detected, it may be necessary for the client to perform the entire activity once again. Thus, it is preferable to check progress as frequently as is feasible, throughout the activity, rather than waiting until the task is completed. Once again, the trade-off between speed and accuracy applies.

Sustained attention and resistance to distraction. It is probably most efficient to manipulate the environment to reduce distractors, whenever possible. Clients may be able to remove material from a large office or common work area to work in a relatively quiet to isolated environment. During counseling sessions, clients' ability to attend to a task can be addressed by providing them with periodic cues from the counselor. These cues can be as simple as giving them a token after a defined time period of sustained attention, or giving them a written prompt to monitor whether they have been maintaining attention. The interval of time between the counselor providing cues can then be increased, or the client can be given more responsibility for self-monitoring of attention lapses and self-reinforcement for paying attention. These procedures of using a reinforcer or written cue to maintain attention to a task can be readily incorporated into the work setting, with the supervisor, job coach, or co-worker trainer providing cues as necessary.

Attention to task can also be increased by providing benefits to staying on task. For example, the tokens used as cues can be given either symbolic or tangible value. On the work site, the client can also be reinforced for maintaining on task behavior by being provided periodic benefits; for example, work breaks can be made contingent on task-performance rather than time contingencies.

Problem solving and organization. Clients can utilize some form of formal problem-solving framework (e.g., D'Zurilla & Goldfried, 1971)[25] which systematically directs the client through a series of cognitive steps. These steps typically include the identification of the problem, review of alternative solutions, selection of a response, and verification of a solution. This procedure is well suited to training interpersonal problem solving within the context of therapy using a variety of social, functional, and vocational examples.[26] It also appears effective to have clients identify potential or actual problems from their daily experience, and to address these within the problem-solving session.

This procedure may have particular utility in the context of counseling the client about job options, or it may be expanded to involve the client in the discussion and evaluation of specific work behaviors and interpersonal behaviors on the work site. Particular attention can be given to having the client identify both the short-term *costs* and *benefits* to a particular solution, as well as considering the personal and social costs and benefits.

Completion of work in a timely fashion and the ability to carry out work without prompts or excess supervision.   Self-management techniques and checklists may be taught to increase a client's independence and ability to perform a regular schedule. For example, Shafer (1987)[27] used a self-instructional procedure with a client who had difficulty completing a series of janitorial tasks independently. This procedure involved four steps: asking questions of himself about what tasks need to be completed; answering the questions in the form of a rehearsed series of statements; guiding the performance with follow-up statements related to individual task analyses and requirements; and self-reinforcement with praising statements. The same procedure can be supported with written prompts, checklists, visual graphs, portable tape recordings of the self-statements, or other cues to support clients' cognitive functioning.

Social judgment and communication.   Inappropriate social behaviors and poor social judgment may be related to lack of knowledge or ability to perform necessary social skills, lack of awareness about one's own behavior, difficulty recognizing social cues and feedback, or reduced behavioral self-control. Clients should be given immediate, direct feedback regarding their social interactions within the counseling session, and therapists are obviously a powerful model for appropriate social behavior. It is important to assess the client's available social skills as a possible source of poor work behavior. For example, one woman was frequently late or absent from her job without notifying her supervisor, who became increasingly irritated by her lack of respect and "not caring" about her job. In counseling, she appeared motivated and cooperative, valued her work experience, and recognized the difficulties that her poor attendance was causing. She revealed that her transportation was often delayed in picking her up, but did not know what to do when that happened. As an interim intervention, at least, the client was taught to notify her supervisor by phone whenever her ride was more than 15 minutes late.

Role-playing can be used to develop a repertoire of appropriate social responses. It is often helpful for the patient to have a sample of well-practiced and routine responses for different social situations, e.g., greeting and responding to supervisors and co-worker, waiting for appropriate moments to speak or make non-disruptive interruptions; responding to suggestions or criticisms, and so on. Having a rehearsed selection of responses will often reduce social anxiety and help to avoid the emotional consequences of difficult social interactions as well. Inappropriate social behaviors may be related to difficulty in understanding the intentions or meanings of others' actions. Clients can practice forming interpersonal hypotheses to explain the behavior of others, and validate these with the therapist.[28] Self-monitoring of inappropriate verbalizations or social behaviors can be conducted through diaries, notebooks, or checklists and can be an effective means of providing the client with feedback about his or her behavior and training social skills. The majority of problems with social and work behaviors exhibited by clients with traumatic brain injury are probably related to cognitive and behavioral deficits resulting from the injury, rather than being intrapsychic or conflict-based. Treatment, therefore, needs to assist clients to recognize and compensate for their deficits to reduce these symptoms.

Group work and group therapy

Group psychotherapy can be a valuable component of counseling for clients with traumatic brain injury, and may be especially valuable in facilitating the process of socialization by which the client learns to relate with others and assume roles within the family, community, and society.[29] Group therapy provides a means to place the client in a social situation, and therefore, more closely approximate the demands of real life. This can serve to reduce clients' social isolation, and at the same time demands a broader repertoire of social and interpersonal behaviors. The group situation can be an effective means of having clients experience the effects of their injury on their social behavior, and the effects of their social behavior on others. Within the group, socially appropriate behavior needs to be maintained while inappropriate behaviors are diminished. Experience with group processes of turn-taking, compromise, personal risk-taking, self-disclosure, and other social skills is readily transferred to work and daily living situations. The use of structured exercises, homework assignments, and videotaped feedback are applicable in the group setting, and can be of assistance in helping clients develop awareness and ensuring that generalization of skills or behaviors is actually occurring.

For some clients, sharing experiences with other persons who have traumatic brain injury is a powerful form of alleviating their sense of alienation and demoralization. Clients may particularly benefit from feedback from other clients regarding their cognitive limitations, emotional reactions, and social behaviors. In may instances, clients are able to accept this peer feedback when they are unable or unwilling to accept feedback from a psychotherapist, rehabilitation professional, or others. Support groups may be structured around specific vocational issues, e.g., job seeking or job placement. For clients who seem unable to appreciate or tolerate the group process, it is possible to have more structured, psychoeducational or discussion groups in which clients can ask questions about specific medical, neuropsychological, vocational, or other factual topics. This can be effective in promoting a gradual expression and sharing of clients' experiences and feelings.

Clemmons and Fraser (1991)[30] have identified a vocationally supportive format for group work with clients with traumatic brain injury that contains four aspects. These are a climate of acceptance, a bridge to reality, a sharing of the patient's world, and a climate of appreciation. This basic model of group interaction is important in the development of a positive attitude toward group interaction by both clients and counselors, and may be seen as a precursor to developing the therapeutic conditions discussed by Yalom (1975).[31] In using group interactions to foster vocational activities, there may be a combination of psychoeducational, behavior change, and support group emphases. According to these authors, the utility of group interaction to the vocational re-entry process includes the following:

1. Reinforcement of program goals
2. Evaluation of social functioning
3. Opportunity to evaluate a spouse, parent, or friend as a resource
4. Presentation of didactic information regarding head injury and related issues
5. Building an *esprit de corps*, reviewing the progress of different group members within the vocational program
6. Specific problem solving within a job-related context

The format for these groups first involved an initial 10-15 minutes of general social interaction, followed by a formal topic presentation supportive of vocational progress (e.g., conversational skills, effective job interviewing, effects of and avoidance of alcohol and drugs following TBI, or safety concerns following a TBI). Another 10-15 minutes socialization break was followed by 40 minutes of facilitated discussion, role-plays, exercises, etc. This educational structure is less threatening for some clients who would otherwise shun psychotherapy interventions and is generally well-received. Although a minor portion of the group, two to three significant others usually attended, and were sometimes very helpful during role plays and general assistance in group interaction. The psychoeducational program was available to each new group of 15 clients coming to a University of Washington vocational services demonstration projects sponsored by the Rehabilitation Services Administration.[30] Typically, about nine clients took advantage of the group (attendance was encouraged but not mandatory).

The format and content of these groups appear to work well, with clients, spouses, parents, and friends included in the group. This type of group requires an active and well-organized therapist. This structure with breaks for socialization seems to work particularly well. In some instances, separate groups for clients and significant others may allow difficult emotional issues to be more readily addressed. Lauer-Listhaus (1991)[32] describes a group structure for significant others only. It was a structured, educational format which was very useful in engaging difficult family members and providing valuable information regarding care in traumatic brain injury, or assistive intervention. This psychoeducational group began with very basic topics such as services available through the state brain surgery association, medical complications of a TBI, and psychiatric problems and behavioral management issues through final sessions facilitated by the group leaders that focused on grief and loss with discussion of effective coping strategies. Ten, $1^1/_2$ hour sessions were offered over several months, the first half of each session being didactic followed by question and answer — a somewhat similar format to that developed by Clemmons and Fraser (1991).[30]

Prigatano (1986)[2] and others have utilized *cognitive group therapy* and group psychotherapy, as well as ancillary educational group for relatives of clients. Cognitive group therapy is a form of group therapy that focuses on improving social perception and facilitating effective communication. Initially, the purpose of the group is to increase the level of self-awareness of cognitive strengths and weaknesses. It is the responsibility of group members to provide appropriate feedback to one another. This process frequently generates strong emotional reactions, but is necessary to help individuals form realistic perceptions and expectations.

Group psychotherapy, as utilized by Prigatano's group, is a more traditional therapy directed at the emotional and motivational disturbances associated with brain injury. The focus is on helping clients recognize and modify the various types of personality and affective disturbances that are associated with traumatic brain injury. The initial aim of group psychotherapy is to help clients break down their sense of social isolation, and help them identify their emotional difficulties. A long-term aim is to have clients be able to identify their own emotional reactions in a group setting and to deal with these collectively in a productive way. As underscored by Pepping (1998),[33] through the group, both self-awareness and interpersonal skills can be developed. These factors can be critical to work and also successful independent living. Dr. Pepping emphasizes that successful people are aware of their deficits and get along well with others.

It may be helpful to have a prepared list of topics for discussion at different sessions or points in a session. These might include what group psychotherapy is all about, common emotional reactions and personality changes after brain injury, the catastrophic reaction, body image, self-confidence, and feelings concerning work and having to go back to work at a lower level.[2] Mangel (1990)[34] has developed a structured format for group psychotherapy based on the various topics suggested by Prigatano (1986)[2] and others, which includes a framework for facilitating client discussion and feedback.

Process considerations in the provision of group psychotherapy in TBI rehabilitation

There are a number of factors in the effective provision of group psychotherapy. These are discussed in more detail in the article by Pepping (1998)[33] A summary of this author's guidelines with additional considerations includes the following:

1. Two facilitators are ideal for this type of group, ideally a male and female, to provide complementing perspectives; more effective role playing; supportive, leadership energies; and more responsive timely

intervention with group members, and as referenced by Pepping (1998, p. 41),[33] a "healthy second family experience."

2. Group size should allow for a reasonable and substantive mix of individuals, but can get unwieldy if it exceeds eight — regular attendance is required or strongly encouraged.

3. The therapist(s) must be very active and often directive — gauging an individual's emotional readiness for input, and often, the best neuropsychological modality through which to reach a person both cognitively and emotionally (e.g., often visual or sensory).

4. Many sessions can have a specific educational theme and be somewhat didactic, but the therapist(s) looks for opportunities to reflect an individual's perceived feeling state and relate it to others in the group or evoke potential feelings from others on an issue. Simultaneously, the facilitator(s) must be sensitive to potentially explosive situations and assess when not to intervene with a group member, or carefully use a "sandwich technique" style of approach (i.e., facilitator presents a positive reinforcing statement about a member, then some feedback which could be taken negatively or might be emotionally difficult to absorb, followed by a positive closing statement).

5. To be a more effective process, modalities might change to optimally meet the needs of group members: role playing (often video taped), practice in conversational or social skills, drills in using verbal compensatory techniques, use of pre-group mood-setting music, metaphors ("why might you feel like a low battery?"), projective drawings to reach feeling states, use of stories to underscore issues in adjustment, etc. In essence, to be effective, a group leader(s) might stretch the bounds of creativity, and realize the need to be flexible.

6. Despite the use of different group process modalities, the group leader(s) must be attuned to modulated pacing, the underscoring and repetition of important themes that are group relevant (e.g., personal self-awareness, awareness of emotion and mood management, or necessary social/interpersonal skill development), and the importance of not covering too many topics or themes in a session.

7. Therapist(s) will be more effective if they can share their own emotions and personal reactions, as this can be ideal modeling and increases their credibility in the group. Group leaders with good senses of humor and resilient egos are particularly important in this arena — especially when working with a group of younger male clients not prone to self-disclosure or personal openness even prior to their injury.

Due to limited funding and time for rehabilitation activities, group psychotherapy in TBI rehabilitation programs is not always readily available at rehabilitation centers. There are also obviously a number of challenges for the therapist involved in this effort, and not every therapist is up to the task. Nevertheless, New York University, Oklahoma Presbyterian Hospital, and some local brain injury associations are able to support this type of service. Other sites have shown the benefit of this type of psycho-therapy service — hopefully it can be utilized more often in the TBI reha-bilitation effort. Its use is a function of funding, organizational commit-ment, and the availability of enthusiastic and skilled therapists.

Conclusions

In general, it is wise to consider the counseling relationship as a model of clients' interactions with the rest of their social and vocational environment. The therapist needs to be sensitive to a client's cognitive, behavioral, and emotional limitations and adjust the counseling interactions accordingly, while maintaining an attitude of caring and emphatic understanding. The therapist also needs to be able to confront the client, challenge the client, and foster the prospect for change; acceptance of the client does not mean acceptance of all of the client's behaviors.

The therapist additionally needs to be able to promote the application of skills and behaviors outside of the treatment session. The functional appli-cation of therapy appears to be enhanced when training is prolonged, the client is given increasing responsibility for his behavior, and feedback about the utility and appropriate application of his behavior is provided. The failure to maintain an appropriate therapeutic distance constitutes a common therapeutic error. When addressing a client's cognitive deficits we have relied on a simple rule: when the client succeeds, provide less assistance; when the client fails, provide more assistance. In similar fashion, when the client appears to have difficulty engaging or participating in therapy, the therapist needs to approach the client and increase the client's involvement within therapy; when the client appears to be overly reliant on the therapist and has difficulty applying the lessons of therapy outside the treatment environ-ment, the therapist needs to increase the client's autonomy and involvement outside treatment.

If return to work or school does represent a return to normality for clients who have sustained traumatic brain injury, then the therapeutic relationship and interactions represent a powerful vehicle for that return. Together they provide clients with opportunities for new learning and experiencing, for developing awareness about their presumed and actual abilities, and for confronting — and hopefully reducing — the discrepancies between their assumptive world and their daily reality.

References

1. Price, P. and Baumann, W.L. (1990). Working: The key to normalization after brain injury. In D.E. Tupper and K.D. Cicerone (Eds.), *The Neuropsychology of Everyday Life: Issues in Development and Rehabilitation*. Boston: Kluwer Academ-ic.
2. Prigatano, G. (1996). *Neuropsychological Rehabilitation After Brain Injury*. Balti-more: The Johns Hopkins Press.

3. Pepping, M. and Roueche, J.R. (1990). Psychosocial consequences of significant brain injury. In D.E. Tupper and K.D. Cicerone (Eds.), *The Neuropsychology of Everyday Life: Issues in Development and Rehabilitation*. Boston: Kluwer Academic.

4. Chelune, G.J., Heaton, R.K., and Lehman, R.A. (1986). Relation of neuropsychological and personality test results to patients' complaints of disability. In G. Goldstein and R. Tarter (Eds.), *Advances in Clinical Neuropsychology*, (Vol. 3). New York: Plenum Press.

5. Fordyce, D.J. and Roueche, J.R. (1986). Changes in perspectives of disability among patients, staff and relatives during rehabilitation of brain injury. *Rehabilitation Psychology*, 31, 217–229.

6. Fordyce, D.J. (1999). Counseling issues and strategies after brain injury. Presentation in the Traumatic Brain Injury Rehabilitation Internship, University of Washington, Seattle, March 10, 1999.

7. Cicerone, K.D. (1989). Psychotherapeutic interventions with traumatically brain-injured patients. *Rehabilitation Psychology*, 34, 105–114.

8. Uomoto, J. (1997). Psychotherapy for clients with neurological disorders. In *Directions in Clinical Psychology*. New York: Hatherleigh Press, 1997, Volume 8, Lesson 5.

9. Faust, P., Guilmette, T.J., Hart, K., Arkes, H.R., Fishburne, F.J., and Davey, L. (1998). Neuropsychologist's training, experience and judgment accuracy. *Archives of Clinical Neuropsychology*, 3, 145–163.

10. Cicerone, K.D. (1987). Overcoming obstacles to change. Presented at National Head Injury Foundation Sixth Annual Symposium, San Diego, CA.

11. Beutler, I.E. and Clarkin, J.F. (1990). *Systematic Treatment Selection*. New York: Bruner/Mazel.

12. Dunbar, J. (1980). Adhering to medical advice: A review. *International Journal of Mental Health*, 9, 70–87.

13. Lobitz, C. and Shephard, K. (1983). Effect of compatibility on goal-achievement in patient/physical therapist dyads. *Physical Therapy*, 63, 319–324.

14. Galano, J. (1977). Treatment effectiveness as a function of client involvement in goal-setting and goal-planning. *Goal Attainment Review*, 3, 1–8.

15. Crosson, B., Barco, P.P., Velozo, C.A., Bolesta, M.M., Cooper, P.V., Werts, D., and Brobeck, T.C. (1989). Awareness and compensation in post-acute head injury rehabilitation. *Journal of Head Trauma Rehabilitation*, 4, 46–54.

16. Pine, F. (1985). *Development Theory and Clinical Process*. New Haven: Yale University Press.

17. Meichenbaum, D. (1985). *Stress Inoculation Training*, New York: Pergamon.

18. Weinstein, E.A. and Kahn, R.L. (1955). *Denial of Illness*. Springfield, IL: Charles C Thomas.

19. Helffenstein, D.A. and Wechsler, F. (1982). The use of Interpersonal Recall (IPR) in the remediation of interpersonal and communication skill deficits in the newly brain injured. *Clinical Neuropsychology*, 4, 139–143.

20. Kazdin, N. (1974). Reactive self-monitoring: The effects of response desirability, goal setting and feedback, *Journal of Consulting and Clinical Psychology*, 42, 704–716.

21. Bandura, L. (1977). Self-efficacy: Toward a unifying theory of behavior. *Psychology Review*, 84, 191–215.

22. Deaton, A.V. (1986). Denial in the aftermath of traumatic head injury: Its manifestations, measurement and treatment. *Rehabilitation Psychology*, 31, 231–240.

23. Alexy, W.D. (1983). Perceptions of deficits following brain injury: A reply to Roueche and Fordyce. *Cognitive Rehabilitation*, 1, 4–23.

24. Stapleton, M., Bennet, P., and Parenté, R. (1989). Job coaching traumatically brain injured individuals: Lessons learned. *Cognitive Rehabilitation*, 7, 18–21.

25. D'Zurilla, T.J. and Goldgried, M.R. (1974). Problem solving and behavior modification. *Journal of Abnormal Psychology*, 78, 107–126.

26. Foxx, R.M., Martella, R.C., and Marchand-Martella, N.E. (1989). The acquisition, maintenance and generalization of problem-solving skills by closed head injured adults. *Behavior Therapy*, 20, 61–76.

27. Shafer, M.S. (1987). Supported competitive employment: The use of self-management programming in the follow-along process. *Journal of Rehabilitation*, July/August/September, 331–36.

28. Leftoff, S. (1983). Psychopathology in the light brain injury: A case study. *Journal of Clinical Neuropsychology*, 5, 51–63.

29. Diehl, L. (1984). Patient-family education. In M. Rosenthal, E.R. Griffith, M. Bond, and J.R. Miller (Eds.), *Rehabilitation of the Head Injured Adult*. Philadelphia: F.A. Davis.

30. Clemmons, D.C. and Fraser, R.T. (1991). *Vocational re-entry of the traumatic brain injured: A demonstration project*. Unpublished manuscript, University of Washington, Department of Neurological Surgery, Seattle.

31. Yalom, I. (1975). *Theory and Practice of Group Psychotherapy*. New York: Basic Books.

32. Lauer-Listhaus, B. (1991). Group psychotherapy for families of head injured adults: a psychoeducational approach, *Counseling Psychology Quarterly*, 4:4, 351–54.

33. Pepping, M. (1998). The value of group psychotherapy after brain injury: a clinical perspective. *Brain Injury Source*. Winter, 14–49.

34. Mangel, M. (1990). Structured group psychotherapy with patients with traumatic brain injury. Presented at Rebuilding Shattered Lives: Third Annual Conference on Traumatic Brain Injury, Woodbridge, New Jersey.

chapter three

Use of assistive technology in vocational rehabilitation of persons with traumatic brain injury

C. Gerald Warren, MPA

Introduction: A brief history and definition of assistive technology

In 1988, Congress passed an important piece of legislation affecting the opportunities of persons with a disability, the Technology Related Assistance for Individuals with Disabilities Act of 1988 (PL 100-407). This law provided program support to states to assist them in establishing statewide assistive technology programs for all individuals with a disability. The definitions that evolved during the development of that legislation helped clarify the role of technology in meeting the needs of persons who are disabled.

Research and development addressing equipment for persons with a disability began in earnest in the late 1960s, with the emergence of the field of bioengineering. In 1973, the Rehabilitation Engineering Centers were established and federally funded to perform the pertinent research and development. In 1986, the Amendments to the Rehabilitation Act of 1973 (Public Law 99-506) required the use of rehabilitative engineering in the development of an Individualized Written Rehabilitative Plan for clients of state vocational rehabilitation services. This action truly launched the era of service delivery for assistive technology.

Until 1988, the terminology *rehabilitation engineering* was commonly used to refer to any high or low tech services being provided to individuals with disabilities. During the development of PL 100-407, the terminology and definitions concerning this field were further clarified. The term *rehabilitation engineering* is now most commonly used in rehabilitation research and development, while the term *assistive technology* is used when referring to delivery of equipment or technical services to persons with disabilities. There are two main reasons the rehabilitation engineering nomenclature has given way to the term *assistive technology*. First, many of the people who are providing or receiving technical services are not involved in rehabilitation programs, but may be in special education, health maintenance, services to the elderly, etc. Therefore, the *assistive* adjective is generally applicable. Second, when services are being provided to persons with disabilities, it is technology as opposed to engineering which is being delivered. The term *engineering*, therefore, was more appropriately changed to *technology*.

In the development of the new law, assistive technology was also defined as technology designed for and used by individuals with the intent of eliminating, ameliorating, or compensating for functional limitations. Further definition divides the definition of the technology into two parts: an *assistive technology device* is any item, piece of equipment, product or system, whether acquired as a retail item, a modified retail item, or a customized one, that is used to increase, maintain, or improve the functional capabilities of individuals with disabilities. An *assistive technology service* is defined as any service that directly assists an individual with a disability in selection, acquisition, or use of any assistive technology device.

In 1990, Public Law 101-336, The Americans with Disabilities Act (ADA) declared that individuals with disabilities have fundamental rights of equal access to public accommodations, employment, public transportation, and telecommunications. The stipulations of the law eventually established the civil rights of people with disabilities to have society recognize its obligation to facilitate attainment of their life objectives, particularly in the workplace. The law not only addressed the need to assure accessibility to buildings and structures, but made provision for consideration of the reasonable accommodations that could be made to allow a person with a disability to accomplish the essential functions of a job.

The law defines a qualified person with a disability as one who is capable of performing the essential functions of a job with *reasonable accommodation* on the part of the employer. Under this definition, persons with disability who would not be able to perform essential job elements following an attempt at reasonable accommodation are not protected under ADA legislation. At this writing, the term *reasonable accommodation* is not legally defined in the statutes, and disputes regarding this issue are settled in court.

Application of appropriate assistive technology is clearly the methodology by which the accommodations are accomplished. The responsibility for implementing the accommodations is generally attributed to the employer. However, state vocational rehabilitation funds are often used to perform a site evaluation and in some cases, implement accommodations where it is clear that the resources from the employer are not available — often a small business or a non-profit agency which cannot support the expense. In some cases, special rehabilitation project funds or the person with the disability may have funds to pay for the accommodation. The law does not define the term *reasonable accommodation*; the definition is found in the courts who determine whether an employer's claim of undue hardship is valid. Congress continues to amend the original Rehabilitation Act of 1973, Public Law 93-112, and with each amendment the level of recognition of assistive technology's role in supporting persons with disabilities, particularly in the workplace, continues to grow.

Why use assistive technology with persons experiencing a TBI?

In vocational settings, the major functional limitations encountered by persons with traumatic brain injuries fall into the categories of *mechanical* and *process* limitations. The mechanical limitation relates directly to difficulty in physically accomplishing work activities. The process limitation refers to the inability of cognitive functions (e.g., to attend to, organize, sequence, and evaluate the result of work activities).

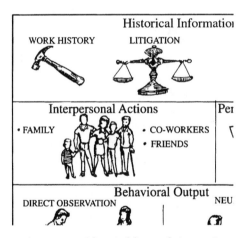

Figure 1   Computer software provides problem-solving assist.

If we were to step back and look at what technology brings to our modern work world, we find there has been a tremendous technological impact on both mechanical and process concerns. This is particularly true in production or service-oriented environments. Coincidentally, we find that the residual abilities of persons with traumatic brain injury are often quite useful in production or service-oriented work environments (Figure 1).

The assistive technology that can be used to overcome mechanical limitations is often simple and inexpensive. Simple, inexpensive solutions can also be effective in solving process problems. It has been shown, however, that in dealing with complex process issues, the logic available in computer technology may significantly contribute to a person's ability to function. Such applications need to be evaluated to assure that they are appropriate and cost-effective.

Use of simple assistive technology is often pivotal to the development of a vocational plan or a productive workstation. Often the process effort in identifying an appropriate intervention can be more involved and costly than the intervention itself. The consultation and evaluation phase of the process, conducted by experienced clinicians, is often the most important phase of a successful intervention.

Secondary effects of applying assistive technology

Assistive technology applied in a vocational setting may be the first time a person with a brain injury is offered assistance that does not appear to be typically clinical. The intervention is often empowering; it can allow the person to amplify his/her effect on the world. It can contribute significantly to the ability to be productive and to be more effective in activities other than mobility, self-care, or activities of daily living.

By the time a vocational objective is addressed in a rehabilitation program, clients have usually been well counseled and have a generally positive "can do" attitude. It is not uncommon to initially experience need denial on the part of a client. Clients may have difficulty participating in an intervention not presented appropriately. The benefits of an intervention need to be properly introduced and described to each client. Enlisting a client's aid in developing an intervention can be important to gaining acceptance. Staging an intervention and introducing it a little at a time can help to achieve acceptance and higher levels of function.

There are often significant behavioral changes following assistive technology interventions. Clients often exhibit newfound pride and feel empowered, as they begin to use their new tools. The intervention may cause dramatic changes in productivity and can foster a positive, competitive attitude and new inspiration. This is generally a desirable outcome. In some settings, however, it can both positively and negatively affect group dynamics which can foster undesirable behavior in some co-workers. Some interventions will involve co-workers' education and advocating their support of the new activities.

Assistive technology can also threaten the sanctity a person sometimes finds in disability. Occasionally, individuals may express very positive attitudes toward returning to work but covertly believe that because of their limitations, they will never be able to do it. Suddenly, a technical intervention may eliminate the barrier they felt protected them. The rehabilitation assistive technology intervention can provoke a wide variety of behaviors or issues that had not previously surfaced within the rehabilitation process. The rehabiliation professional should realize that the implementation of assistive technology is a time during which additional social or counseling support may need to be provided. A psychologist/neuropsychologist or rehabilitation counselor may need to be involved in this discussion and clarification process.

Impaired functions that limit vocational outcome

There are a range of functions that may be impaired following a brain injury. The salient areas of functional concern are reviewed below.

Sensory-motor integrity

Sensory and motor performance can be critical factors affecting competent job performance. Consider the five senses of sight, sound, touch, smell and taste. Each is controlled by a specific area of the brain and injury to these areas can cause loss or impairment of these senses. There are obvious limitations associated with a person's inability to hear. These are not only associated with general communication, but in the workplace can have significant impact on safety. Sounds may indicate the need to pay attention, the presence of danger, or alarm.

There are also obvious limitations due to loss of sight or low vision which will interfere with the worker's productivity or effectiveness in the work setting. For individuals with a brain injury, however, there is also the high probability of visual-perceptual difficulties. When working with an individual who has documented visual difficulty, it is extremely important to know exactly what that individual can see. This often requires evaluation by a professional who is skilled in functional visual evaluation rather than one who would provide just a standard opthomologic examination. Some senses, such as smell or taste, are not usually important to most jobs considered for this population. Smell, however, can often provide an early warning of airborne toxic substances or smoke.

Reduced or absent sensation in the fingers and hands can be a significant problem for those involved in production work and assembly. Problems are encountered by workers required to manipulate small parts if they have difficulty feeling or distinguishing shapes by touch.

Reduced control of motor function has significant impact on a person's ability to perform in a job requiring any level of physical activity. Accuracy, fine dexterity, and speed of performance as well as sufficient motor strength/balance must be evaluated and correlated with the specific job function if a person is to perform tasks adequately. This can involve very careful job analysis.

Attention and concentration

Attention involves awareness of important stimuli occurring in a person's environment. Concentration means the ability to focus and maintain attention and not be distracted by other stimuli for a period of time. Persons with brain injuries often find it difficult to concentrate or focus attention on one task for a significant period of time. This concern is often complicated by the presence of distracting stimuli occurring in their school or work environments. These difficulties are a major concern as they can interfere with learning, acquiring new job skills, and basic job performance (accuracy and productivity), as well as safety.

Memory

Memory for recent or past events may be one of the greatest concerns when considering vocational objectives. As with attention and concentration, memory deficits significantly affect the person's ability to acquire and retain the knowledge and skills necessary to maintain employment. They may restrict the complexity of tasks to be performed as well as the range or number of activities the person may perform.

Memory is commonly divided into verbal and nonverbal components. Verbal memory is generally evaluated by determining a person's ability to remember a short passage or lists of words which have been read aloud, and measuring both immediate and delayed recall of information. Nonverbal, or visual-spatial, memory is typically evaluated by measuring a person's ability to recreate simple line drawings or geometric figures presented on a stimulus card. Again, the protocol frequently involves measures for immediate and delayed recall of the stimulus figure. More subtle aspects of memory assessment include consistency, the ability to categorize and store information, response to retrieval cues, and so forth.

It is very important in vocational planning to identify both strengths and problems in memory function. A person may have problems with verbal memory, while visual-spatial or nonverbal memory is chiefly intact. In more severe cases of brain injury, most aspects of memory function can be impaired. Even in these cases, many individuals can become functional for work or independent-living activities with an appropriate cueing system. It is necessary to understand residual memory strengths when developing an assistive technology approach to aid job performance.

Language function

Knowing the level of language function is very important in achieving vocational goals. Language function assessment may be as elementary as determining levels of vocabulary, as well as the more complex assessment of receptive and expressive language. Receptive language refers to one's ability to understand language input, either spoken or written. Individuals with receptive language problems may misinterpret, or simply not understand spoken or written information. Even relatively subtle difficulties in this area can greatly impair communication and a person's ability to follow directions consistently.

People with expressive language deficits, conversely, may understand language input, but have difficulty expressing their thoughts to others.

Again, these deficits may involve written language, spoken language, or both. A person with traumatic brain injury may have both expressive and receptive language problems. Language-related problems are frequently, but not exclusively, associated with left-brain injuries.

Visual-spatial abilities

Visual-spatial abilities are complementary to the area of language function. Visual-spatial abilities are generally associated with the functions of the right cerebral hemisphere and involve such abilities as form recognition and spatial relationships. Deficits in these abilities can influence a person's capacity to perform a wide variety of critical job-related tasks. These generally include tasks requiring mechanical ability, scanning and assessing part-to-whole relationships, sequencing physical activities such as assembly, etc. Visual-spatial problems are often less obvious than language deficits. Even when language is intact, visual-spatial deficits create organizational and problem-solving limitations which can affect job performance, especially in the trades.

Cognitive efficiency

Cognitive efficiency is a complex function which involves the integration of a number of brain-related functions. These include the ability to sequence tasks, to quickly process information, to change tasks or carry on parallel activities, and to work in the presence of distractions. Many minimum-wage positions, such as fast-food service workers, require the person to switch rapidly from one task to another, or to combine several tasks. A person with lowered cognitive efficiency is likely to become confused, make errors, or become bogged down when multiple tasks must be performed in rapid or random sequence. Individuals with deficits in this area are often quite capable of performing repetitive tasks or jobs composed of linear tasks which can be easily chained together.

Executive functions

Executive function involves a variety of abilities used to monitor and administer life activities. These abilities vary widely even in people without brain injury. Persons with brain injury may have increased difficulty with abilities such as planning and prioritization. Evaluative questions concerning executive function include

- Is this person able to plan for activities and decide which are important and which are not?
- Can the person initiate activities and get going on a plan of action?
- Can a person continue to prioritize activities?
- What is the individual's ability to problem solve or resolve issues that do not have an obvious next step?

- Can they make appropriate decisions and/or learn from mistakes?
- Self-regulation is an important executive function. Can a person monitor and evaluate actions and make the appropriate changes with environmental feedback?
- Is the person able to adapt when plans need to change?

We have been discussing brain function capabilities that can act, often in combination, to significantly influence a person's ability to function in a vocational setting. Appropriate executive functioning becomes more important with increasingly complex job activity. The brain functions we find impaired in persons with head injury are often amplified or exaggerated functional difficulties that can be easily found in a number of general population members.

Behavioral concerns in the workplace

Issues of integration

In planning an assistive technology intervention within an organizational setting, the first thing that must be identified is who the players are, who will the intervention affect, and who will influence the intervention. The obvious focal point is the participant; however, we need to consider the other individuals who by their awareness or involvement can influence the success of an intervention. The people to consider as part of the team are the links to the payor or rehabilitation agency. The vendor clarifies the immediate supervisor, co-workers, or other workers who will come into contact with the person receiving the intervention. The roles of a potential job coach or other job site mentor and the involved vocational rehabilitation counselor are pivotal. There are, on occasion, union representatives and advocates who also directly or indirectly become involved and their potential influence must the recognized.

A clear understanding of management's expectations of the person must be established. This should include employee appearance, performance, and productivity goals. The perception of each player's role must be explored or understood to help assure a positive outcome and to avoid "surprises." Implementation of accommodations needs to follow the same basic principles used in performing quality job development when the same set of players is usually encountered.

In order to assure system-wide support and compliance with the implementation of the accommodation program, it is important that there be demonstrable management support and understanding of the objectives involved in an intervention. This is generally accomplished easily with an introduction or outline of the proposed plan presented to management in a positive manner. Such a presentation must emphasize that the plan has or will be developed with concern and awareness for the need to minimize the impact of any intervention on the company. There is frequently considerable sensitivity among managers who fear the cost of accommodating a worker with a disability. If the company is paying, the benefits of a tax deduction or credit need to be outlined for the company manager and administration. Data from the President's Committee on Employment of the Handicapped (President's Committee, 1990)[3] indicate, however, that the majority of the modifications cost less than $500. This is also the time to emphasize how the proposed program can enhance management and corporate images. Some display of support from management in the form of written or unwritten policy should be evident to all the players.

Another important objective, if possible, is to identify a champion or mentor who supports integrating an individual with TBI into the work environment. This may initially be a specific counselor, job coach, or rehabilitation advocate who has been involved in developing the work opportunity. It is also important to identify early on, a potential supervisor or other worker (e.g., paid or unpaid co-worker) who has the energy and time to take on a mentor/advocacy role. Whoever this person is, care must be taken to assure this advocate's productivity is not compromised.

The champion or advocate needs to be trained and made fully aware of the technology that is being applied and, if appropriate, to know how to trouble-shoot it, modify it, and when and how to call for help. The client should also be encouraged to take responsibility and be able to ask for help as needed.

At times, an intervention may make it possible for a person with a severe disability to perform a task, but it may not make that person sufficiently productive. Interventions need to be rigorously evaluated to assure that the work being performed is of sufficient value to sustain the individual worker's role. A partially successful intervention, artificially sustained, can produce a prolonged, agonizing situation for the worker and/or his employer.

Obviously, any intervention provided for the disabled worker cannot be disruptive to the work pattern of that individual, or those around him or her. In all cases, we must avoid or minimize the intervention that may interfere with space requirements, make things more awkward for other workers, introduce excessive noise into the environment, or interfere with other workers who may need to use the same space or equipment on other shifts. All of these factors must be considered as we focus on meeting the needs of the worker with a disability.

Risk management

Risk management is a very important consideration when applying assistive technology in the workplace. To a large extent, this involves the safety of the client and co-workers, but it should also extend to minimizing the liability of the employer. Care must be taken to consider the implications of the workers' roles in interacting with customers or the public, and the possible influence their work may have on the performance and reliability of a product or service.

Assistive technology can also be used to reduce risks to individuals with head injuries in the workplace by controlling behaviors such as roaming; helping them pay attention to the tasks at hand; and by providing alarms, protective guards, or equipment that contribute to safety. Introducing technology that increases the independence or capability of the individual within the workplace can also introduce new risks. This is particularly true when the individual is given expanded freedoms and mobility or when power tools are introduced into the client's work setting. Use of power tools by persons with brain injuries should be carefully evaluated and scrutinized. It is particularly important to analyze risk when equipment or mechanisms are used which produce significant mechanical advantage or powerful forces in their operation.

At times, there needs to be concern for the safety of others, as illustrated by the example of the worker whose task it was to use a hammer to pound T-nuts into blocks of wood that were components used in a cabinet-making operation. When this worker became frustrated and/or enraged, he had a propensity to throw his hammer, which in fact, in a ricochet, slightly injured a co-worker. Consequently, this hammer was, replaced by an eighty-pound arbor-press that was bolted to the table (Figure 2). The worker used a crank handle on the press to seat the T-nuts, eliminating the need for the hammer and its potential for becoming a dangerous missile in the workplace. Any number of risk management interventions can be just this basic.

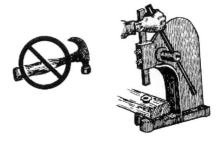

Figure 2   Risk management: changing work tools.

Maximizing the clients' residual knowledge and skills

During the vocational and neuropsychological evaluation, data are often revealed that indicate the strengths and fields of interest that an individual may have had in the past. It is very important to delve into the premorbid knowledge and skills that the individual had in the workplace, in hobbies, general interests, and academic pursuits. As discussed by Dr. Uomoto in Chapter one, evaluations are often too focused on deficits. Assets must be identified and leveraged through the use of assistive technology, which can allow a person to apply residual knowledge, skill, and interests in a vocational setting. The following case studies represent a range of assistive technology examples used to maximize client residual capabilities:

Example 1

Problem: Cortical blindness and limited ability to sequence activities.

Intervention: Modification of fabric-cutting table to properly control equipment and placement of tactile cues for making measurements.

BR who had worked in a large furniture-manufacturing firm as an upholsterer incurred a head injury that resulted in limitations to the number of steps he could complete in sequence. He also had a significant degree of cortical blindness.

Working with his former employer, a fabric-cutting table was modified to provide a method for the individual to perform routine fabric cutting. A jig system was developed to provide a guide and ensure safe control of the fabric knife. Tactile cues were placed on the surface of the table to give information on the size of the material being cut. This opportunity allowed the individual to work in a familiar environment and for him to use his residual knowledge of materials and the process. His co-workers, who knew him prior to his accident, supported him. All this contributed significantly to his comfort and motivation and very successful employment.

Example 2

Problem: Loss of short-term memory and receptive language.

Intervention: Modification of order-entry system reports that provide the location of items in warehouse.

RW, at 19 years old, had a well-developed knowledge of auto mechanics through his hobby of restoring "muscle cars." His injury in a high-speed auto wreck left him with the inability to initiate and sustain a sequence of activities; this deficit was combined with short-term memory and receptive language difficulties.

He was, however, able to work filling orders in a parts department for a diesel engine and heavy machinery parts supplier with the aid of assistive technology. The report function of the computerized inventory and order-entry system was modified to provide him with a printout, which indicated not only part numbers and prices, but also part names and coded locations in the warehouse. By association, he knew the part by name. When he saw the part, he was able to find it in the warehouse using a coordinate system that was set up using signs with letters of the alphabet to locate the row of shelves in the warehouse, and numbers to define the shelf or bins that held the parts or equipment. Using this method, he was able to reliably retrieve parts and participate in filling customer orders. His reliance on this method appeared to diminish over time and he may indeed not need it in the future.

Example 3

Problem: Moderate ataxia of upper extremity and limited duration of attention.

Intervention: Used computer technology to establish home-based music business.

DS was a very talented musician prior to an accident that left him relatively intact cognitively, but with significant motor ataxia, dysarthria, and a limited attention span. He was unable to use his instrument, but did retain his complete knowledge of music theory.

By attending a school of music, he was able to demonstrate his ability to compose and orchestrate through the use of the school's computer technology. Using a mouse and keystrokes he operated the software and hardware for developing computer-generated music. This allowed him to perform the act of putting notes on paper and then producing the sounds. Using the school's recording equipment in conjunction with the computer, he produced demonstration tapes that received a high degree of acclaim and recognition in the industry. He was able to gain state rehabilitation agency support to equip himself with appropriate software, a computer, and studio recording equipment. He has pursued self-employment in the area of producing studio-ready compositions for commercial and industrial video presentations. He performs this work in his home studio, pacing himself to maximize his productivity.

Example 4
Problem: Ataxia of upper extremities, poor visual field tracking.
Intervention: Use of a computer and software to set up a home-based business in which his wife became a co-worker to support his limited motor function.

RW has moderate ataxic and has vision control difficulty, which limits his ability to change visual fields. He has an MBA and was formerly financial manager of a medium-size business. He was also quite capable of comprehending and operating spreadsheet and bookkeeping software. He was capable of operating the computer to perform analysis and report preparation, but could not enter data at a rate that would be considered a good use of his time. RW wanted to be self-employed, offering administrative and financial services to small businesses in the industrial parks near his home. He was provided a computer, appropriate software, and re-training. Arm supports were provided to improve hand stability and assist in keyboard function. Copyholders were used to strategically place source documents adjacent to the computer screen to reduce his visual tracking difficulties.

His wife took a refresher keyboarding course to support him by doing the data entry. RW assumed an "executive" role, supported by the skills of a person with good motor and visual control. This is an example of job restructuring and co-worker assistance.

In some cases, using a person's residual skill or knowledge can be limited because they cannot achieve the appropriate rates of task accomplishment. At times there may be no technology to overcome physical limitations, particularly in keyboarding. Resolving these issues may involve a division of labor or job restructuring so other workers can perform tasks requiring rapid physical activities.

An emphasis on computer technology and electronics to augment function

Milton and Wertz (1986) described a set of techniques they called *compensatory strategies* which have been demonstrated to make substantial contributions to functional ability, particularly when applied in supportive employment programs. These strategies are appropriate when a person has reached a plateau and exhausted the ability to show functional gain from rehabilitation interventions. The person can now benefit from external sources of support to compensate for specific cognitive limitations, such as memory, as illustrated in Figure 3.

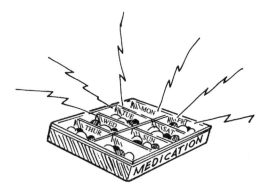

Figure 3 Memory aids: a medication reminder.

Compensatory strategies, which include memory notebooks, lists, and written schedules, have regularly been used to assist in memory and executive functions. These strategies are very useful for individuals who have the ability to remember or can be cued to use them. This system must be maintained and organized and works best when the person is involved in linear or a linked series of activities. These strategies are usually implemented manually and require the person to function at a fairly high level or assistance must be provided to maintain the program. The greater a person's need for such approaches, the more complex the strategies may become, and this results in a much higher "overhead" in maintaining and supporting a program. The manual strategies are passive and do not provide active cueing of the user or an opportunity for the program to be interactive.

Use of computer technology

Computer equipment and software, which have been developed for busy, able-bodied individuals, can be used to augment the theories and methods that are used in manual compensatory strategies. Use of such software and equipment can contribute to much higher levels of function for individuals with head injury residuals and be carried out with less overhead or support costs than manual methods. This is accomplished by using the programming features of off-the-shelf software.

Such approaches offer the advantage of being able to develop a structured or automated *input* capability that can be used by an individual to control the system themselves once the process is set up. Such systems can also provide a well-structured *output* that clearly and consistently organizes information. This can improve the individuals' ability to comprehend cues or instruction.

If the software application being used is programmable, it offers the opportunity to create strategies with multiple facets. By using simple logic statements, an interactive scenario can be established that has the user respond to inquiries displayed on screen. The display might ask if a task has been completed. If the answer is no, the program can redirect the person to perform the next appropriate step in the sequence of activities or give an alternative action. If the answer is yes, the instructions for the next task or action are displayed. This type of program can provide control over sequencing and completion of multiple tasks. Speech output, audible cues, or alarms can be programmed into such a system to stimulate the user.

To use this technology successfully, a person must have reading and receptive language skills, and be motorically capable of operating the equipment (computer) independently. Operating a computer can be done through the use of alternative input methods. These would include modified keyboards or switch-activated systems that substitute for keyboards when interfaced through augmentative communication equipment.

To benefit from computer-based technology, the user must have the ability to respond to cues and have an attention span sufficient to accomplish the sequence of activities being prompted. When such strategies are intended to assist a person with attention, concentration, or memory deficits, we must verify their ability to take advantage of the cueing or prompting that can be provided by the technology. This should be determined in a simulation or trial activity prior to embarking on a program that is likely to have significant expenses involved.

The advantages of using electronic/computer technology over a manual compensatory strategy are that multiple audio or visual alarms can be used to stimulate responses, and input strategies and structural output can be designed to assist a person in performing multifaceted or branching activities. The disadvantage of using such equipment is the expense involved, which includes software and hardware costs, plus the cost of developing and maintaining a program and the training of participants that is required. Continued follow-up is also needed to ensure maintenance of ongoing programs and any implemented changes so that the benefits of the expenditure are realized.

The equipment used to accomplish some of these compensatory strategies can range from sophisticated hand-held calculators to pocket or palmtop computers (Figure 4), portable computers commonly referred to as Personal Digital Assistants (PDA) integrated with laptops, and/or desktop equipment. The sophisticated calculators and palmtop computers can be used primarily for scheduling activities. Many have sophisticated multiple alarm systems in the software that can be combined with a note pad function for display of prompts. The market for this type of equipment and the features offered has been volatile due to rapid changes in technology and industry competition, but it has begun to stabilize because the PDA is becoming much more useful to business and salespeople. These devices are essentially small personal computers that have standardized software memory and programming capability. Some models allow information to be uploaded, i.e., moved from the palmtop to the desktop computers, and downloaded, moving information from a desktop computer into the memory of the palmtop computer.

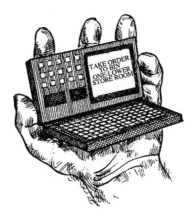

Figure 4   A palmtop computer.

Notebook/laptop computers are the next step up in computational capability and operate at the level of low-end desktop computers and are constantly being refined. Software can be integrated into systems used in office or home environments and will help support a person with limited memory at the level of executive function that they may need in the work, educational, or home environment.

Augmenting academic and vocational activities

In this section, the discussion assumes cognitive status has plateaued. The methods discussed here can support an individual who is trying to deal with permanent, non-remediable deficits that may be interfering with the ability to participate in mainstream training or work. These may be deficits in cognitive function or in performance of physical activities. The difficulties experienced by a person with a brain injury are often just an exaggeration of the difficulties that can be observed among non-brain-injured persons.

Executive administrative function

For the purpose of executive functioning in an academic environment, there are several areas in which persons with a brain injury have notable difficulty. The first is the organization or management of the activities that are required in the training or academic program. These activities usually are related to time management and, to a great degree, involve scheduling activities: A person may have difficulty allocating time to accomplish tasks, keeping appointments, or being adequately prepared for class.

Verbal and written recapture function

A second area of major difficulty can be a client's ability to receive, retain, and process information. The most common difficulty occurs when the rate and/or volume of information being conveyed to the person become overwhelming. Retention and use of information are highly dependent on a person's receptive language functions and the ability to organize and process information for retrieval. This function significantly influences a person's ability to participate in an academic program.

Verbal and written expressive function

Participation in an academic program also requires that students be able to output information that reflects an increase in their knowledge and/or skill base. A common problem is the physical inability to present the information, either in verbal or written format, due to motor problems. This may be combined with executive functioning limitations, which include the inability to compose appropriate output, to format and/or configure it in an acceptable manner, and to have it be accurate or correct in spelling and grammar.

When considering interventions in any of the above areas, it is very important that the applied technology will not interfere with potential cognitive or physical gains that may later be made by the person. Introducing the support technology can be a great concern for the clients and their advocates, even though it has been determined clinically that the individual has truly plateaued. The introduction of any form of assistive technology to aid a student or worker must be done with sensitivity, and demonstrated to be a tool to increase the capability of productive daily activity or quality of life.

There are a variety of methods for assisting people to cope with problems involving academic achievement. Using computer technology to assist a student in academic pursuits should be considered, because it may be able to contribute to solving a variety of problems for that individual. When appropriate, a computer can be used to augment the standard techniques of using printed schedules or memory books. Major advantages include the clarity that can be achieved in both input and output format; use of interactive cueing, color, or highlighting; help functions, and audible cues or alarms.

Common software that is used to assist busy able-bodied individuals keep their lives in order is appropriate for use by a person with a brain injury. There are a variety of personal scheduling software programs that are easy to use and combine time and place control with notation or note-taking functions that correlate with the scheduled events. Some have multiple alarms to serve as cues.

These schedulers are usually memory-resident software that are automatically invoked when the computer is turned on, and they run concurrently with other software running in the background. These programs allow the user to toggle or transfer in and out of the scheduler with minimal key strokes or be able to rely on alarms which will go off as set. These features can be used on most desktop or portable computers, and several personal digital assistants have scheduling modules. Such aids can assist clients with memory and executive functioning deficits (organization skills, sequencing, etc.).

When dealing with individuals who have good keyboarding skills and receptive capability, taking notes on a portable computer during a presentation can be a feasible but, at times, difficult activity. It can be done using appropriate outlining software or a flexible and easy-to-use word processor. Types of software categorized as personal information managers employ artificial intelligence techniques to allow input of free-form information into a database and retrieval with English language queries. Sometimes called *random information managers*, these tools can be powerful in dealing with the organization of unstructured information. A quiet keyboard on the computer avoids the potential problem of annoying noises in the classroom.

Difficulties in being able to receive information, either from written or verbal sources, can be enhanced through the use of assistive technology. Collecting spoken information through the use of tape recordings is often suggested; however, it must be remembered that it usually takes as long to listen to information as it did to record it. This, in effect, doubles the person's time commitment. There are two ways of overcoming this problem. The first option is to use a tape recorder with speech compression playback, which allows a person to play back a recording at a minimum of double the speed it was recorded. This equipment usually has a frequency compensation function to make the speech more intelligible. This may not be a good solution for a person having comprehension problems due to rate of speech, but it can also be used to quickly scan the content and then re-listen to segments of interest at normal speed. A second alternative involves very small digital recorders that are very useful for making "verbal notes" that can be easily retrieved. The capability of these recorders is limited to a few minutes, but a series of comments only a few seconds long can successfully assist a person with short-term memory problems.

In the area of language and, in particular, composition, there are several tools to assist a person who is having difficulty finding the right words, organizing them, and spelling them correctly. Word prediction software could be useful if the individual is capable of finding the first few letters of a word. By entering the prefix of a word, a program displays the potential words in a window on the screen. The words may even be displayed and ranked in the order of probable use in that person's vocabulary. Word finding can be aided with the use of thesaurus and/or dictionary functions that can be called upon by using a "hot key" to turn the function on and off. Spellcheckers can be used on line, i.e., checking each word as it is being typed, or applied to a completed document to show errors and provide alternative spellings which are usually displayed in a window on the screen. Grammar checkers can be used to evaluate text and identify grammatical errors and provide alternative ways of constructing sentences. Spelling- and grammar-checking functions are features of standard word-processing software.

Software that provides a "macro" capability can be used to reduce the number of keystrokes required to enter repetitive information or text into a computer. This type of software allows one to easily "program" or set up the computer software to recognize a few unique keystrokes (usually 2 or 3) that will produce a long series of keystrokes automatically when the unique keys are activated. An example might be using two keystrokes to produce the salutation of a letter written frequently to the same person.

When using computers to assist a person with a brain injury, easy access to the programs is essential. Software should be organized on the computer so that after the power is turned on, the person is automatically taken to a point which allows access to whatever tools are desired through menus or icons, symbol selection, or automated help functions.

Other electronic aids

Some research has been conducted into the effectiveness of using computers in task guidance activities. Kirsch et al. (1988)[1] at the University of Michigan are one group that has conducted these studies. Their findings suggest that interactive cueing can facilitate task performance. In one study, four subjects with traumatic brain injuries who performed part of a janitor's job using either computerized task guidance or written directions were evaluated. Two of the patients consistently improved their performance when using computerized task guidance versus written directions. Generalization to competitive employment, however, was not established.

Parenté and Anderson-Parenté (1990),[2] in their writing on vocational memory training, discuss the fundamentals of using electronic cueing devices, dictation tape recorders, auto-dialing telephones, signaling devices, car finders, and checklists. They discuss the use of electronic phone dialers that are carried in one's pocket. These are used to store numbers for visual feedback, and some models when acoustically coupled to the telephone can be used to auto-dial. There are wristwatches (e.g., made by Casio and Seiko) that have alarms, which can be used to alert or remind an individual to participate in a pre-established activity.

For individuals prone to losing things due to attention or memory issues, an electronic sound-emitting device can be attached to the item and the sound triggered by a variety of methods including a whistle, hand clap, or activation of a small transmitter. A similar approach can be used by a person who, on occasion, doesn't remember the location of his automobile in a parking lot.

The electronic equipment used in such applications are often gadgets that are marketed to busy or forgetful able-bodied persons. The market for these items is volatile and specific models of a product may not be consistently available for purchase or replacement. If such equipment is used and it has the potential for becoming a key element in a person's functional regimen, it is important that the product or a similar one will be available if broken or lost. Continuity of these aids is an important consideration.

The sources for much of this equipment are stores and mail order catalogues, such as Radio Shack, Sharper Image, Brookstone, and Dak, among others. Further information on a wide range of products can be accessed through ABLEDATA, the nation's leading source of information on products for disabled persons (ABLEDATA: Newington Children's Hospital, 181 East Cedar Street, Newington, CT 06111, phone (203) 667-5405, web site: www.abledata.com). Another source of actual job-site accomodation information/assistive technology strategies is the Job Accommodation Network (JAN) at West Virginia University (phone 800-342-5526 and web site: www.csuchico.edu/abilcon/DR/gen/janbbs.html). More recently, JAN, the service sponsored by the President's Committee on Employment of People with Disabilities is also consulting on self- or home-employment strategies/accommodations.

Electronic/computer technology can be used very effectively in a variety of employment settings. Representative work-related applications are described in the following case studies.

Case Study 1

Vocational Impairment:	Worker with problem-solving deficits wanders into dangerous areas in search of people to help him.
Implementation:	Remote-controlled flashing light is used to summon help.

TW is a 26-year-old male who, as a result of a head injury in an automobile accident, had significantly reduced executive functioning abilities. He did retain moderately good motor control, muscle strength, the ability to learn and follow a short list of specific instructions, and he was highly motivated for work. TW was placed in a job at a very large paper-recycling operation. His major task was to empty very large wire baskets of paper from pallets into an industrial shredding machine.

Several accommodations were made to improve the physical process of his emptying a basket and maintaining his safety. One major difficulty arose as the result of the shredder being located in a visually isolated area. When TW had completed emptying a basket, his strong motivation to continue being productive caused him to wander in search of a fork lift driver to remove the empty basket and provide him with a full one. Having TW wandering around in the facility was quite dangerous, as there were several forklifts moving materials about the warehouse at a very high rate of speed. The forklift drivers could hear each other and used their horns, but they could not hear TW who would appear at unexpected places in the warehouse. TW's need to wander was resolved by providing him with a radio frequency transmitter, the size of a TV remote control (Radio Shack). The receiver module was a switch that was used to turn on and off a large flashing red light mounted high on a post in the center of the warehouse. Whenever TW was in need of a forklift driver to replenish his supply of paper, he would press the button on his transmitter to turn on the beacon, and a forklift driver would respond at his next opportunity. TW would then turn the beacon off. He was very pleased with his new system of empowerment, and was also kept from harm's way.

Case Study 2

Educational Impairment:	Student having difficulties with high-school program due to impaired executive functioning.
Implementation:	Provided a computer system that integrated a palm top and a desktop computer.

MS, a 14-year-old male, suffered a gunshot wound to the head. He retained reasonable cognitive capabilities related to language skills, new learning ability, and memory retention. He was able to resume his high-school education in a mainstream environment. MS was, however, severely limited in his executive functions, (e.g., self-regulation) and had difficulty with time management. He often failed to be at the right place at the right time. Without a great deal of family assistance, he was unable to organize his work and/or assignments to be completed on time.

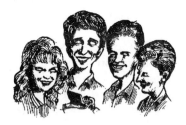

Figure 5   Social benefit of the palmtop computer.

As he resumed more activities outside the home, he was often embarrassed because his support system did not extend into the community. Because of his relatively high level of performance in most functions, his peers did not understand his periodic confusion and disorientation and on occasion would tease him. He began to withdraw and to make even more judgement errors, such as leaving school before it was over or not showing up for counseling or tutoring.

After a series of training sessions and with the help of his family, MS was able to learn to use a palmtop computer the size of a wallet. It had clock/calendar scheduling and notepad functions with multiple alarms. He learned to use the equipment to create and respond to daily and weekly schedules. At any time he could discreetly refer to his computer and query it for current or upcoming activities that had been input. He could also set reminding alarms throughout the day or week. On hearing the alarm, he was referred to the "note" that he had associated with the alarm to retrieve the instruction or activity details to be carried out.

MS uses a desktop computer at home to perform his academic assignments, and he carries the palmtop computer with him to school. It provides him with appropriate prompts and cues about time and place, and he can also use it to capture limited amounts of information on the calendar and notepad. He is also able to load files from the palmtop into the desktop computer, and combine them with the note-taking capabilities and scheduling functions that he maintains on that computer.

The use of the palmtop computer at school not only increased his functional capability, but generated a good deal of interest, and a degree of prestige among his peers that helped him further stabilize emotionally. The social reinforcement value of such a tool for many adolescents should not be overlooked.

Case Study 3

Vocational Impairment: A woman with quadriplegia and lack of verbal speech (although using augmentative communication equipment).

Implementation: By interfacing her communication equipment with a personal computer, she had the opportunity to enter the work force.

RL is a 32-year-old woman who had a brain stem aneurysm, which resulted in quadriplegia, severe spasticity, and loss of vocal capacity. After a long rehabilitation process, RL became independent in her mobility using a powered wheelchair with chin control. She mastered communication through an augmentative communication system, which was mounted on her wheelchair (Light Talker by Prentke-Romich; Shreive, Ohio) (Figure 6). RL operated the communication equipment using a small optical receiver which was mounted on her glasses. By directing the receiver at locations on a matrix of cells on the Light Talker, she was able to select letters, words, and phrases, which could be displayed on a screen or spoken through the equipment using synthesized speech.

Once she had mastered the augmentative communication system, it was evident that RL was very intact cognitively. After completing her medical rehabilitation and overcoming major bouts of depression, she became quite aggressive about her desire to do something productive. The most obvious

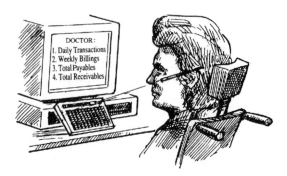

Figure 6 Use of a light talker to operate computer.

technical avenue for RL for environmental interaction was through the use of a personal computer. RL was obviously unable to operate a personal computer with a keyboard; however, the communication equipment she owned could be interfaced to a computer and become its keyboard. With these possibilities in mind, the next step was to determine vocational opportunities that were appropriate for her to pursue and could be accomplished through the use of a computer.

RL had been a receptionist in a dental office for many years prior to the injury. This information triggered a search for personal computer software that could be used to manage dental clinic operations. At this point, a commitment was made to provide RL with a personal computer, appropriately configured to run business software. The interface between her communication equipment and the computer was also purchased. By using a radio frequency link between her communication device on the wheelchair and the computer, RL could be independent in approaching or leaving her computer, i.e., her equipment did not have to be physically connected.

RL then began the process of becoming knowledgeable in the basic operation of a computer, and the specific software for management of a dental office was leased. After a very short period of time, it was easy to recognize that RL was completely able to operate the software package intended to manage a dental office. She became very proficient in the use of the computer for a variety of standard applications.

Efforts to place RL in a dental clinic facility in the rural area in which she lived failed, and RL did not have the support systems necessary to allow her to move to an urban setting to pursue this further. Therefore, RL continued to become proficient in the use of her personal computer and learned to use a computer-based voice mail system. This system allowed her to operate an answering service for the academic staff of a local community college, an alternative which still provided her a reasonable level of job and life satisfaction.

Case Study 4

Vocational Impairment:	Dysgraphia and visual dyslexia causing poor work performance and loss of job.
Implementation:	A portable computer and software provided tools for retraining.

GL, a 26-year-old male, received a severe concussion in a bicycle accident. He achieved complete motor recovery, and good cognitive function, but exhibited symptoms of dysgraphia (difficulties in writing) and some visual dyslexia. GL resumed his work as a coordinator of sports programs and promoter of running events and marathons. For several years, he was able to work, although he had a good deal of difficulty with his written communication. At times, he would simply avoid it. These difficulties resulted in several disputes and negotiating difficulties. He finally was forced to resign as a director and promoter of the activities, due primarily to poor written communication that frequently resulted in personal misunderstandings and confrontations.

Further neuropsychologic evaluation demonstrated his ongoing difficulty with dysgraphia and some visual dyslexia. The dysgraphia made it difficult for him to write longhand or draw, and the visual dyslexia interfered with reading and interpreting. His verbal language reception and expression were excellent.

GL decided to pursue a graduate degree, and with the use of a portable computer, was able to overcome the challenges of note-taking, i.e., capturing information and producing reasonably constructed information. His use of computer software and equipment and development of good keyboard skills accomplished this. He was trained on how to take notes in real time, by using a dictating and manual transcriber for practice. A portable computer with very quiet key action was selected for use in class and he was able to take down essential information during the lectures using word-processing software. He took these notes and transferred them to a database or constructed new text files. He could augment the information, and construct output in the form of reports, papers, and other documents. He used the dictionary, thesaurus, spellchecker, and grammar-checker built into the software. The grammar checking program allowed him to examine his text for standard grammatical errors and to look at options for improved ways to express himself in sentence construction. With this software and equipment, GL is well on his way to completing a Masters degree in Public Affairs. He will continue to use this technology as he pursues a career in public policy.

Case Study 5

Vocational Impairment:	Gross spatial and path-finding activities.
Implementation:	A vehicle-based navigational system was implemented.

DM had the physical and cognitive ability to safely drive a vehicle. Prior to his injury, he had a commercial driver's license. He also exhibited particularly good personal qualities for work in the often demanding activity of providing quality personal transportation alternatives for persons with disabilities.

DM was hired as a driver for a personal transportation operation. It soon became evident, however, based on his inability to keep a schedule and the frequency with which he became lost in the city, that he now did not have the capacity to reliably navigate throughout the community.

Personal vehicle-based navigation systems are an emerging technology which uses micro computer technology to combine data from a global position satellite (which identifies the location of an antenna on the face of the earth within plus or minus 3 meters) with digital graphic representation of city street maps. This provides the user with a display, which not only shows one's present location but can also provide visual and auditory direction for the pathway between any two locations that have been input into the processor.

This equipment is sold as an accessory to be installed in personal transit vehicles. To use the equipment, the user inputs the current location and the desired location. The processor computes the route, which can be modified. Based on the system's direction, the user is given cueing that indicates upcoming intersections and provides information on the appropriate turns to be made to follow a designated route. Should an error be made and the user get off track, the processor recalculates the route to bring the user back onto the desired course.

This technology was purchased and installed for DM and it gave him the opportunity to be a successful driver throughout a major metropolitan area. The cost of this technology and intervention was approximately the cost of a personal computer that might be used to support a person with a disability in an educational or business context.

Adapting work environments

Work environments present two major challenges for persons with brain injury. The first involves coping with the cognitive complexity of activities or series of tasks. The second relates to having the motor control and/or strength required to physically perform the activities.

When placing a person with a head injury at a work site, it is very important to perform a task analysis of the work to be accomplished early in the process. The most critical (important) and time-consuming tasks deserve special attention. Counselors and job placement specialists need to be diligent in their efforts to identify any functional impasse as early as possible and seek a possible solution through the use of assistive technology.

Understanding the workflow and influence of associated operations

In performing these analyses, there are many aspects of the work environment that need to be explored and understood, beginning with management policies, production schedules, and expectations for output or production. Each step required to complete a task must be identified as the work flows through the workstation. It is important to understand the process by which the worker receives products and/or materials. The details of how each task is physically accomplished, and finally, what happens to the material or product as it leaves the workstation deserve attention. Resolving a person's work-related impairments often occurs by introducing minor procedural modifications.

Analyzing and modifying the specific tasks to improve performance

In many work settings, particularly in supported employment, clients are often capable of performing the tasks, but can only do so at low or marginally productive rates. Job coaches and trainers are constantly challenged with the need to increase productivity and meet minimum standards for continued employment. In such instances, it is important to develop performance data that can be captured through traditional time and motion studies of the tasks or individual activities involved in the job. It is also important to demonstrate which elements of the task are taking an inordinate amount of time, and to "baseline" performance so that the effects of an intervention can be documented and evaluated. Observing and defining each element of the task or the task sequence will reveal the task(s) or activity that needs to be modified or eliminated. These analyses may lead to reorganization of the process, providing materials or tools for the person, or changes in the sequencing of the tasks involved. This analysis should precede the introduction of direct-task modification or use of additional equipment.

Ergonomic considerations to improve speed and endurance, and avoid fatigue

When a client is involved in physical activities that are highly repetitious, are conducted for prolonged periods of time, or require a specific physical effort to accomplish, the ergonomics of the work setting are important to consider. Attention must be paid as to how the client interacts physically with the workstation or equipment. When work activities are being performed by a person with a physical limitation, the pattern or sequencing of the activities may significantly affect the speed and accuracy of work activity. The person's endurance and fatigue are directly influenced by the level of effort that must be applied in performing the activities.

Individuals with physical limitations are challenged to accomplish certain tasks, and certainly, being able to perform an activity can be a major triumph for such a person. However, considerable attention must be paid to whether the task is being accomplished at an appropriate rate and if the person can continue to perform the activity for prolonged periods of time, without fatigue. Fatigue may occur in individual muscle groups, i.e., finger flexors, shoulder elevators, elbow flexors, etc. Does the person get a sore or painful neck, shoulders, back, or feet? We must also consider the overall physical impact of working a full shift for an individual. Does the client go home exhausted, sore, and unable to participate in social or leisure activities? Maintaining an energy level balance at work to ensure that there is residual energy for a person to carry out non-work activities is important. This helps to assure successful long-term work and enhance general quality of life.

Case Study 6

Vocational Impairment:	Impaired finger dexterity limited the worker in a critical job task of labeling.
Implementation:	Pre-formatted labels so that special equipment could be used.

LB is an 18-year-old woman, injured in an automobile accident, who has moderately reduced general cognitive function, good upper extremity mobility, and gross hand function, but difficulty with fine motor control and finger dexterity. LB was placed in the packaging and mailing division of a company which responded to magazine coupons sent in for mail-order pet identification tags. In the system, the employee processed information from the coupon to produce a mailing label and manufacture the corresponding pet tag. LB's job was to receive the mailing labels and the tags, correlate the information, be sure that the right tag was with the right mailing label, place the mailing label on the envelope, and insert the coupon and the tag into the envelope in preparation for mailing. She was able to adequately perform the major tasks with the help of a number of bins and hoppers to organize the envelopes, cards, and tags. With her limited hand function, the major problem was peeling the mailing labels from their backing and placing them on the envelope.

As a functional solution, the mailing labels were generated on a computer printer and came to LB in sheets, with three labels across horizontally. Her task was to pick each label off individually and apply it to an envelope. Investigation of the process of producing the labels indicated that the software used to print the labels on the computer could be changed to print the labels in a single sequential strip. This made it possible to use a manual label dispenser into which she could easily load the labels. The dispenser provided labels to LB one at a time, making it easy for her to get the label from its backing and onto the envelope. Work-site intervention for individuals who have experienced a TBI can often have a physical dexterity emphasis vs. higher order cognitive issues.

Case Study 7

Vocational Impairment:	Reduced executive and fine-motor functioning.
Implementation:	A simple tool was developed that allowed the worker with a TBI to perform challenging tasks while his co-worker assumed the easier but more time-consuming activities (example of task reallocation with co-worker).

DU is a 22-year-old male, who had significantly reduced cognitive and executive function, reduced fine dexterity and hand function, but good gross motor capability. DU works on the production line in a running stroller manufacturing plant. One of the jobs involved he and a co-worker assembling handles for the strollers. A handle was placed in a jig, and DU used a hand-drill motor to make a series of holes and then rivet straps onto the handle. This was an easy eight-step sequence that he could perform. His co-worker at the other end performed six steps. Five of them, installing a splash guard, were easy. A sixth difficult one, however, involved attaching plastic trim around the edge of a piece of sheet metal.

The problem identified was that DU could not complete his eight steps fast enough, and he left the co-worker waiting for as much as one-half to a full minute for DU to complete his steps. The initial request was to determine how DU's productivity could be improved for his eight steps. An evaluation of the tasks revealed there were no physical modifications to the jig that would help DU and there was little margin for improving his rate of performance; therefore, the focus was directed to the work being done by his co-worker. DU was not assigned these tasks because he was unable to manage the application of the plastic-edging material to the sheet metal. A relatively simple wooden tool was designed to assist in this step, and he was trained to use it effectively. DU swapped positions with his co-worker, and the new set of work tasks balanced perfectly with his co-worker's efforts to increase the handle assembly production.

Case Study 8

Vocational Impairment:	Worker with severe motoric hand involvement was slow, but also bored with menial tasks in a restaurant.
Implementation:	Capitalized upon her social skills for greeting patrons, with the assistance of an electronic door opener.

ML is a 23-year-old female who uses a powered wheelchair for her mobility, has reduced hand function and cognitive capability, but a bright and cheery personality. She was placed in a local restaurant where her primary tasks were to wrap cutlery in a napkin in preparation for table setting, and to fill sugar, salt, and pepper dispensers. With some jigs built to help accommodate reduced dexterity and balance hand function, she was able to do the tasks but remained quite slow and extremely bored.

It was the restaurant's policy to have an employee dressed in uniform greet the customers as they entered and left the restaurant during mealtime, i.e., 11 a.m. until 2 p.m. and from 4:30 p.m. to 7 p.m. The task was to open the door for the customers, and welcome them or bid them farewell.

ML's demeanor and appearance made her a likely candidate for this position; however, she was unable to operate the front door of the restaurant. Management was approached about the feasibility of ML doing this job with an accommodation. With management concurrence, the assistance of the building owner, and state vocational rehabilitation agency funding, an electric door opener was installed. It not only made the building more accessible, but it enabled ML to sit just inside the door and open it for approaching customers and appropriately greet them. In general, she functioned quite well in the hostess position and enjoyed it immensely.

Case Study 9

Vocational Impairment:	Limited hand function results in not meeting production requirements in stamping and sealing envelopes.
Implementation:	Jigs, guides, and sequencing activities increase client productivity to acceptable levels.

TB, an 18-year-old female, had significantly reduced cognitive function, but was capable of performing serial tasks. She used a powered wheelchair and had functional use of only her left upper extremity.

TB was placed in a firm that produced gaskets under military contract. Each batch of gaskets that was shipped needed to be packaged and individually stamped with the military specification of that particular part number. One of TB's jobs was to stamp an envelope package for each gasket using a self-inking stencil stamp. The elements in the task were as follows: a large stack of envelopes or packages were placed in front of TB, she would pick up the stamp lying on the table, apply it to the package on the top of the stack, put the stamp down, move the stamped package to the pile to her left, pick up the stamp and repeat the process. Observation showed that the greatest time loss was in picking up the stamp and putting it down.

The problem of having to put the stamp down was resolved by building a hopper that would hold the stack of unstamped packages on a two-inch high step or platform on the right side of the hopper. A rubber fingertip was attached to the right side of the stamp. The fingertip protruded below the level of the stamp but would collapse when pressed on. When the stamping action was complete, TB lifted the stamp and used the protruding rubber tip to slide the stamped package off the stack onto the lower level of the hopper. With this modification TB could continuously stamp up to 50 packages without putting down the stamp. These modifications were shown to increase her productivity in excess of 300%.

TB had a second job sealing the envelopes once the gasket had been packaged. This involved introducing the envelope into a machine aperture, which grasped the envelope and pulled it through the heating elements that heat-sealed the package. TB had difficulty with the rate of processing and maintaining the correct orientation of the envelope. A simple sheet metal guide was attached at the aperture. The guide gave TB a target and a solid backstop that kept the envelope in the correct physical orientation and fed it into the machine. This modification, combined with the re-organization and positioning of the materials, again increased her production in excess of 300% and significantly reducing the incidence of improperly sealed envelopes.

Case Study 10

Vocational Impairment:	Worker could not maintain the proper sequence of tasks that were critical to him being productive.
Implementation:	A jig was designed that guided him in performing the activities in the correct order.

DU, whom we discussed in a prior case study, had a second job of performing the quality control inspection on the wheels used in the manufacture of the running stroller. The wheels were shipped in large cardboard boxes to the stroller factory. DU's tasks were to clean the wheel by wiping its rim and tire with a rag and solvent, visually inspect it for the proper tire mounting and spoke integrity, place the correct amount of air in the tire, evaluate the bearing races to determine whether the wheel ran smoothly, and/or to adjust the bearings of the wheel as needed.

In his original work setting, DU would sit in a chair and with his tools and cleaning materials placed on the floor, he would dump out a box of wheels on the floor in front of him, and proceed with his tasks. DU was very capable of performing the individual tasks involved, but he took far too long to complete the work.

In observing the tasks, the problem appeared to be that he did not have a standard sequence he followed, i.e., sometimes he would first check the bearings, spending time adjusting them, only to find a bent spoke which required that he discard the wheel. Second, his tools were often scattered on the floor. He was using wrenches that had double ends of different sizes and had to frequently reorient the tool. To assist DU, a simple wooden workstation was developed which helped him maintain a structured task and use of tool sequence (Figure 7).

The workstation was designed to allow DU to follow a specific prioritized task sequence, i.e., cleaning and visual inspection, pressurizing the tire, and then performing the bearing adjustments. A tool tray was attached to the side of the workstation, which held his tools and cleaning materials, and the air hose was hung so that it was within easy reach. New tools were purchased. These included pliers for opening the box and single-ended wrenches that were also color-coded for sequence. A rolling rack for the good wheels to be stored was placed nearby where he could place the keepers and a large bin was placed on the other side for him to discard the rejects. This type of organizational aid (or structured workstation) is highly

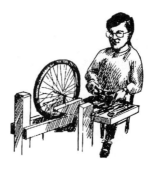

Figure 7 Tool tray organizer resolves sequencing problems.

beneficial for many clients having executive functioning or organizational deficits.

Guidelines for the use of assistive technology

Assistive technology interventions are often characterized as being low, medium, or high technology. In general, the higher the technology level, the greater the cost and this may also be true when equipment is used. However, we must keep in mind that *assistive technology refers to not just equipment*; assistive technology *also includes the methods* by which an objective is reached. The challenge in assistive technology service delivery is to provide the *most appropriate intervention*, i.e., the most functional solution to the person's problem in the most cost-effective manner.

The need for assistive technology continues to grow very rapidly with the recognition of its impact on the lives of people with disabilities. This rapid growth brings forth critical issues of quality assurance. Is the client receiving the most appropriate and safest intervention? Who is qualified to provide these services? To whom and how much should third-party payors reimburse for assistive technology services?

Theoretically, all of these questions should have answers. However, the field of assistive technology is in its relative infancy and as it evolves, so does the development of quality assurance.

The major component of a quality assurance program is the people who perform assistive technology service delivery. They must have the basic knowledge and skills that allow them to adequately achieve the following goals:

- Determine specific functional limitations that can be resolved through the application of assistive technology.
- Develop intervention plans in order to maximize function in all settings.
- Identify available technologies and recommend appropriate utilization.

- Implement the appropriate intervention to achieve maximum function.
- Evaluate functional outcomes of the plan, make appropriate adjustments, and respond accordingly.

To identify individuals qualified to perform assistive technology services, RESNA, the Rehabilitation Engineering and Assistive Technology Society of North America, has developed a credentialing program for assistive technology service providers. RESNA is the primary organization for those involved in the development and implementation of assistive technology and offers specialized training in this area. Eligible candidates may sit for an examination that certifies basic competency to serve the assistive technology needs of persons with disabilities.

There are currently two levels of credentialing; the first is the Assistive Technology Practitioner (ATP), who is most commonly a rehabilitation professional with added competency in the application of rehabilitation technology. The second level is Assistive Technology Supplier (ATS), a person involved in the sale and service of commercially available devices.

The ranks of RESNA-certified service providers are growing rapidly. The chief purpose of certification is to provide the consumer of assistive technology services the opportunity to select providers who have demonstrated a level of competency and pledged to perform their work according to the standards of practice established by their peers.

There is a wide range of straightforward and common-sense interventions performed by clients themselves and/or their advocates that are easily classified as assistive technology. Many of these interventions effectively and satisfactorily meet the identified need. The indicators, however, for requesting assistive technology services are

- When an individual with a disability has functional ability that needs to be augmented or leveraged.
- When a person is highly motivated to increase functioning.
- When you "can't get there from here," i.e., when there is an obvious need to bridge a functional impasse.
- When the "bridge" can be shown to be cost effective.

Assistive technology can truly liberate a person with cognitive or physical limitations. It can be a critical and powerful tool in the rehabilitation and habilitation process and should, therefore, be given appropriate consideration and wisely utilized in meeting the daily needs of a person with traumatic brain injury.

References

1. Kirsch, L., Lajlness-O'Neill, R., and Levine, S.P. (Sept 1988). Improving functional performance of complex activities using two types of interacting cueing systems. *Physical Medicine Rehabilitation, 69*, 714.
2. Parenté, R. and Anderson-Parenté, J.K. (1990). Vocational memory training. In J.S. Kreutzer and P. Wehman (Eds.), *Community Integration Following Traumatic Brain Injury* (pp. 157–168). Baltimore: Paul H. Brooks Publishing Company.
3. President's Committee on Employment of the Handicapped. (1990). *Job accommodation network, evaluation survey.* West Virginia Research and Training Center, West Virginia University, April 1987.

An introduction to vocational evaluation and placement approaches

Robert T. Fraser, Ph.D., C.R.C.

The focus of the remaining section of the text is on providing practical guidance relative to vocational evaluation and placement. Due to the need for comprehensive coverage of the topic, the input of several experts is utilized to give the reader a complete, updated perspective.

Chapter four of this section by Fraser provides a basic framework for vocational evaluation in TBI vocational rehabilitation. It is critical that baseline work access or vocational return goal(s) be established and clarified with the client in a comprehensive fashion. Some of these goals need to be tested as to their viability within the community before a placement effort is undertaken. For the survivor involved in vocational rehabilitation at a residential facility, Brian McMahon, Chapter five, presents an excellent overview of the Affirmative Industry Model through which the residential client can be paid (on- or off-campus) while functional capabilities are being evaluated. Using the Department of Labor 215-hour waiver for non-paid work or other formal volunteer arrangements, other clients can be evaluated within the community with this intermediate level of assessment prior to vocational goal choice.

Once a vocational goal is established, there are a number of placement approaches that can be taken. Chapter six by Fraser and Curl provides an overview to these placement approaches. The work of Rita Curl, Ph.D., in relation to the co-worker as trainer and Paul Wehman on the individual job coach form of supported employment is highlighted among the avenues to placement. As vocational evaluators become more sophisticated in synthesizing vocational and neuropsychological assessment data, they may include a potential approach to client placement as a part of their summarizing vocational assessment recommendations. In some cases, the ecological validity of a particular approach to placement can be assessed while a client is on a community-based job tryout or being assessed within the Affirmative Industry, i.e., test the placement strategy (a co-worker as trainer or the job coach model) during the intermediate phase of assessment. In this manner, the final placement effort using a piloted, often refined approach should be even more successful. Dr. Wehman in Chapter seven describes and encompasses the major components of a supported employment program for survivors of a TBI which should be very helpful for those interested in establishing this type of program. Dr. Wehman has invested significant research and demonstration project efforts in the refinement of the individual job coach model of support.

chapter four

The basis of the placement approach: vocational evaluation

Robert T. Fraser, Ph.D., C.R.C.

In choosing an appropriate placement model for a client with a traumatic brain injury (TBI), a practical first step is generally vocational evaluation or assessment. Without some type of uniform vocational goal-setting procedure, the choice of a placement approach or model can become left to chance. Several articles or chapters in the literature present an overview of the vocational evaluation process in traumatic brain injury rehabilitation. These include work by Fraser (1991)[1] and Chan et al. (1991).[2] The current chapter reviews some of the core issues and describes categories of activity within the vocational evaluation process.

Basic considerations

One of the first of a series of preliminary considerations in TBI vocational evaluation is *who* is conducting your evaluation. It is important that the person conducting the evaluation be knowledgeable about assessment approaches and technologies; have analyzed or have specific job description data relative to the job goal(s) being considered; understand job trends and training opportunities in the local and national economy; be aware of job accommodation methods and utilize assistive technology consultants as necessary; and additionally, understand community resources relative to job securing and maintenance.[2] Perhaps most important, the evaluator should understand the cognitive and psychosocial issues related to traumatic brain injury and have a firm grasp of the neuropsychologic information that needs to be incorporated into the job goal decision and other rehabilitation planning (see Dr. Uomoto's review in Chapter one).

In TBI vocational evaluation, it is also critical that evaluations are tailored to the needs of the individual and that group testing is generally avoided (particularly with individuals having a moderate to severe TBI). Evaluation can begin as soon as the client is able to attend to a task for 20 minutes to half an hour. Commercially available testing and work samples might best be used in such a manner to determine the best learning approach for clients having more severe TBI. There can be less emphasis on traditional normative data and more flexibility in test administration.

Assessment periods may need to be varied due to the effects of fatigue, fluctuations in cognitive capabilities, and reactions to testing such as depression and anger. Many clients will improve dramatically on testing from one to six months, and at one year from injury. Gains still can occur for up to two years, but this improvement is less dramatic.

As emphasized by Chan et al. (1991),[2] the evaluation focus is on the full range of work-relevant behaviors including skill proficiency, work rate, work quality, work endurance, work adaptive behaviors, work values and reinforcers, vocational interests, learning style, and motivation. The emphasis in TBI vocational evaluation is on situational assessment or more of an ecological approach to evaluating the client.[1-3] This can be true not only for clients having a moderate to severe TBI, but also for clients having a mild TBI with post-concussive syndrome symptoms (viz., attentional problems, balance and dizziness issues, memory concerns, headaches, irritability, etc.). Due to the multitude of variables that we are assessing (e.g., cognition, communication skills, other system injuries, behavioral issues) and their complex and variable interaction, the concern shifts to the manner in which these functional limitations may present themselves or interact with the demands of actual work settings. More importantly, what are the assets that enable the client to function, despite presenting limitations — can these assets be identified through a community tryout?

In an ecological systems approach, we observe the client's functioning from several perspectives:[2]

1. There is an attempt to understand behavior by watching how the individual relates to his or her environment;
2. An attempt is made to identify the systems that are most important and troublesome to the individual prior to attempting an intervention; and
3. It is understood that interventions with either the individual or the environment can alter the faulty interaction between the person and the environment leading to maladjustment or poor performance.

Finally, this evaluation can be ongoing and not conclude with an initial job placement. In a study by Fraser, Clemmons, Anderchak, Dicks, and Cook (1990),[4] it was found that two clients on a federally sponsored demonstration project who were terminated by employers at their initial job placements were both soon declared local and regional employee of the month, in two new companies in which they were later placed. Although these events were quite unexpected, the implications of their occurrence are that the barriers identified on the first jobs enabled the job coach and rehabilitation counselors to identify a better person-to-employment setting match in a second placement. Because of the complexity of the disability, some clients' evaluations will continue to be very much an ongoing process for up to a year or more after the initial placement. For some survivors, an initial placement or early placements will be gradual proximations toward a stable job match.

Hierarchical steps in the vocational evaluation process

In traumatic brain injury vocational rehabilitation, one-day vocational assessments for establishing a job goal or specialized assessments involving only a few hours tend to be unusual cases. They are generally not that short unless the client has a milder TBI, a well-focused impairment, or has been involved in a specific skill for years (e.g., welding). For those with more severe impairment, the length of time for the other levels of assessment (transferable skills, short-term or basic evaluation, and long-term evaluation) are generally extended. Due to the complex nature of these disabilities, in addition to the vocational data gathering, it can also be critical to have a considerable amount of input from additional allied health professionals, which may not be as necessary with other rehabilitation clients for whom the injury-related deficits are relatively stable. Transferable skills assessment can require several days to a few weeks; a basic or short-term evaluation generally requires three to four weeks; and an intermediate level evaluation with non-paid or paid work experiences within a facility or the local community can require two to four months before an initial job goal or goals can be established and a placement approach chosen. These procedures are described in a more comprehensive fashion elsewhere,[1,2] but a synopsis of these assessment levels is presented below.

Basic intake and clinical interview

This stage in the process involves an initial comprehensive interview and completion of the intake form by the survivor who is often assisted by family members or a friend. It is a primary step in any of the evaluations to follow, given the value of the information that it can provide. Some rehabilitation personnel conduct this evaluation within a client's home as in a project by Wehman et al. (1990).[5] This includes data collection relative to basic demographics, educational history, prior specialized training, military and work history, psychosocial data to include psychiatric or substance abuse background, availability and types of social support (viz., emotional, job or emergency transportation assistance, personal appraisal, and work and domestic skills advisement). As part of an ecologically oriented vocational evaluation, the assessment of types and availability of social support is particularly critical. Many friends and significant others will abandon a survivor (post TBI) or provide limited support. The survivor and other family members can often assist in the development of job goals. It can also be critical to assess financial status to include types and levels of existing support, specific financial needs (hourly salary within the context of existing subsidies required to enter or re-enter the work force), or any confounding legal processes that may affect the rehabilitation effort. These items need to be established through the intake process, as they are often missed, and it is this lack of information that may later affect rehabilitation planning or placement outcome. A review of all available medical, neuropsychological, independent living, and other data as provided by members of the allied health team is routinely conducted. One review by Zasler (1997)[6] very clearly describes the range of interventions in which the physician, particularly a physiatrist, can be of assistance in maximizing a survivor's functional capacities for work entry or re-entry.

Physical capacities evaluation is often very helpful, particularly as provided by a physical therapy unit or detailed physicians' notes or protocol completion. Thomas and Botterbusch (1997),[7] present a complete Vocational Assessment Protocol (VAP) with a series of nine profiles (including the physical) which can be very beneficial in planning and framing a vocational evaluation or intervention. These profiles are particularly helpful when limited information exists — family members or significant others can assist in clarifying profile information. The last in the profile series actually assists in assessing job search and critical work behaviors in a situational assessment — a more intermediate level of evaluation.

Transferable skills assessment

As in other rehabilitation cases, transferable skills assessment consists of a review of a prior job description and performance standards and whenever possible, a specific job analysis conducted at the prior job site to establish data related to the work's interpersonal and productivity demands, and the quality or accuracy of the required work. Specific work samples are often used to assess the viability of return to work. This can be very important because of the complexity of the variables that can affect performance, especially for those with more severe brain impairment. Computer software searches (e.g., Job Quest* or OASYS**) and traditional occupational resources, such as the Guide to Occupational Exploration (JIST, 1997), can be used to identify other jobs for which the client may be familiar with the tasks or the equipment used. If residual skills cannot be established or another job located within the client's prior company in which he or she has a reasonable interest, the client will enter a basic or short-term evaluation to establish a new job goal(s). Some clients who demonstrate potential for using residual skills in a specific job may move directly into the Intermediate Evaluation phase in which these skills can be further assessed on a community workstation.

* Job Quest, 5805 East Sharp Avenue, Spokane, WA (509)535-5000.
** OASYS (Vertek), 11811 NE 1st Street, #306, Bellevue, WA (425)455-9921

Basic or short-term evaluation

To establish initial job goals or new goals for individuals who cannot return to a prior or related job, this type of assessment, which takes about three to four weeks, is generally conducted. As part of the evaluation, information from other allied health team members and reports from any other recently conducted evaluations (e.g., by the speech pathologist, physical therapist, or occupational therapist) are carefully reviewed. The physical capacities evaluation is often very important for those who have had more severe injuries. Speech is often affected, so evaluators need to be concerned about capacities for receptive and expressive speech, as well as the pragmatics of a client's conversational interactions (e.g., ability to maintain a conversational focus, turn-taking, or voice tone). Other aspects of the short-term evaluation include vocational interest assessment, which may be conducted using picture inventories for those with reading deficits, assessment of work values, and emotional/personality assessment. The Personality Diagnostic Questionnaire,[8] the Minnesota Multiphasic Personality Inventory 1 or 2* and the Millon Clinical Multiaxial Inventory I-III, are examples of inventories utilized to assess emotional or personality concerns. It must be cautioned that the nature of the disability/multi-system impairments experienced by the survivor with TBI, particularly neurological, may elevate scales and exaggerate emotional pathology. Other organic issues can suggest extreme personality difficulties when they are a function of the injury; e.g., a person's lack of self-awareness and self-absorption due to a frontal lobe injury can elevate the Millon's narcissistic scale.

Other areas of assessment include neuropsychological testing and evaluation of worker behavior and performance on relevant work samples. Work samples are often used to determine how an individual may best learn, or to establish potential for job-site training rather than rigidly adhering to evaluation of performance against general normative data. Neuropsychological testing is the cornerstone of the evaluation process in traumatic brain injury rehabilitation. The typical batteries that are used include the Halstead-Reitan Neuropsychological Test Battery,[9] and the Luria-Nebraska Neuropsychological Battery.[10] The McCarron-Dial system, a battery of neurometric and behavioral measures, is often used in the assessment process and sometimes in place of a neuropsychological battery when that is unavailable.[11] In general, due to its neuropsychological skew, the McCarron Dial is very helpful as a core abilities battery in TBI rehabilitation. The author recommends the use of a standard neuropsychological battery or core battery so that the rehabilitation counselor or other staff can develop expertise in understanding the relative strengths and assets of different clients as they relate to employability — this is not to discourage further exploration or additional testing of a specific deficit such as memory issues.

It is important that the neuropsychologist stress assets versus deficits in the neuropsychological assessment process. Due to their training, many

---

* Available through National Computer Systems (NCS), P.O. Box 1416, Minneapolis, MN 55440.

neuropsychologists are overly deficit-oriented in their evaluations. This is certainly important, but vocational rehabilitation counselors need to know the specific existing abilities upon which they can build a vocational rehabilitation effort. This becomes even more important when dealing with limited timelines and/or resources. The vocational rehabilitation counselor must ask specific questions of the neuropsychologist in relation to the client's functioning in certain work activities, and include a job description or ideally, a job analysis with the referral questions.

In relation to academic skills, the Woodcock Johnson Psychoeducational Achievement Battery* and the Adult Basic Learning Exam (ABLE)* are often used. Forms of the ABLE are particularly helpful with those having lesser academic skills, but a desire for post-high-school technical training. Sometimes achievement tests are given untimed, such as the ABLE, to assess knowledge or accuracy vs. speed of cognitive processing which remains impaired. Acimovic, Keatley, and Lemmon (1993)[12] particularly endorse the Woodcock Johnson Psychoeducational Battery for its sensitivity to speed and capacity information processing deficits with individuals having mild injuries. The Woodcock Johnson also appears more sensitive to higher level word-processing and retrieval deficits than some of the lower level aphasia or conversational level assessment batteries. The Weschler Adult Intelligence Scale III (WAIS-III)** is usually administered with the battery.

Because many of the clients who suffer severe brain injury are young and have no significant work experience or well-developed interests, it can be just as important to establish their work values or reinforcers (i.e., what elements of work such as outdoor, a job close to home, etc. may be important to them). Some clients may need exposure to a number of work areas before specific job goals can be targeted. A community job coach or placement person may be appropriate for helping them gain exposure and clarify goals through tours of work sites and a range of job activities — a very valuable agency fee-for-service activity.

The basic evaluation should end with the identification of specific job goals, steps in the continuum to job placement that may be necessary (e.g., what will happen next in an intermediate community-based level of evaluation), barriers that may require intervention or compensation (to include assistive technology consultation as necessary), and if possible, identification of a job placement model, or the identification of clients who require continued vocational exploration because a job goal has not yet been defined. It must be emphasized that further vocational exploration should be intensive and not approached casually, because time is an important commodity to the often anxious client and if work exposure does not happen under the monitoring of the vocational rehabilitation counselor or job coach, it often never will. More information on the use of an *assistive technologist* in traumatic brain injury vocational rehabilitation can be found in Chapter two of

* Available through Riverside Publishing, 425 Spring Lake Drive, Ptasca, IL 60143-2079.
** Available through the Psychological Corporation, 555 Academic Court, San Antonio, TX 78204-2498.

this text by Warren. A specific outline for completing a basic level of evaluation is found in Fraser (1991) (see Appendix A).[1]

Intermediate evaluation

This level of evaluation uses community work experience sites to further determine whether an individual can achieve a specific job goal, or whether the goal needs to be modified and refined. Situational assessment is the most important aspect of evaluation for those with moderate to severe injuries. For example, work experience sites that have been used within the University of Washington and private sector rehabilitation programs within the Seattle area include diverse hospital job sites, university work sites, work experience sites within federal agencies, work sites within community non-profit organizations, and work sites within the private sector. The federal agency work experience program, described in Chapter 306: 11-2 of the *Federal Personnel Manual*,[13] can still be referenced in dealing with federal agency representatives — although program terminology has changed. Despite this work being unpaid, federal agencies can offer work assessment opportunities in diverse sites, particularly in urban areas, and a number of these experiences may convert into permanent job appointments.

The U.S. Department of Labor (1993) has provided a waiver (see Appendix B) which enables individuals with disabilities to work within the private sector on an unpaid basis for the purposes of vocational explanation, assessment, or training. There are a number of contingencies to the waiver (e.g., the worker on a try-out does not displace other workers or give the company an immediate advantage over others), but it allows the individual the opportunity to try a job for up to 215 hours in a private sector position — five hours for vocational exploration, 90 hours for vocational assessment, and 120 hours for vocational training.

If the individual moves to a different tryout position within a company, the 215 hours again become available. This waiver allows realistic assessment of a rehabilitant's capacity to perform any job. Many of these tryouts convert to paid work in a relatively short amount of time. Workers' compensation coverage can be provided by a monitoring rehabilitation facility (e.g., Goodwill) or the State Vocational Rehabilitation Agency.

Private for-profit traumatic brain injury rehabilitation companies with residential programs have developed separate nonprofit employee-leasing companies or have actually added clients to the payroll to pay them and cover workers' compensation insurance while evaluating or training them in landscaping, housekeeping, food service, and other jobs around a facility. In some cases, these individuals are being paid as workers within area businesses while they are being evaluated or trained. These procedures are described in the discussion of an Affirmative Industry model by McMahon in the following chapter.

With increasing severity of injury, it can be critical to perform a job analysis, which includes such information as data relative to specific task activity, production and accuracy criteria, and necessary interpersonal behaviors, or lack thereof at the community work site. In some cases, once the vocational rehabilitation counselor or job coach has framed the necessary data to be gathered, client performance can be monitored and recorded by the job site supervisor or a co-worker. In other instances, a job coach will be needed not only to record necessary data, but also to train the client in specific tasks, cue the client, recommend compensatory strategies, and educate co-workers relative to the client's specific brain-related deficit, such as a specific type of memory deficit. Goals of the evaluation are established relative to the identification of a transition point at which the vocational emphasis can move from evaluation to choice of a placement approach. In order to gauge progress, evaluation meetings are scheduled on a weekly or biweekly basis and information is shared between the vocational staff member, supervisor, and the client and/or significant others. In some instances, a company co-worker or supervisor vs. an agency staff member may replace the job coach in this function. See Chapter six for further discussion of the co-worker as trainer model. Without the community-based intermediate level of assessment, the actual placement approach for many individuals with moderate to severe injuries can be difficult to determine. This, however, can also be the case for individuals with mild injuries complicated by complex post-concussive symptoms.

Summary

This discussion has reviewed the diverse issues in traumatic brain injury vocational evaluation, pertinent knowledge areas for the vocational evaluator, the importance of an ecological perspective within the evaluation, and descriptions of the different levels of evaluation. It is critical that uniform goal-setting procedures of this type are utilized so that staff can develop an expertise with individuals having different levels of injury severity and associated difficulties. Throughout this evaluation process, there is an emphasis on moving to a situational or more ecologically oriented assessment and refining job goals as expeditiously as possible.

References

1. Fraser, R.T., Vocational evaluation. *Journal of Head Trauma Rehabilitation*, 6, 46, 1991.
2. Chan, F., Dial, J.G., Schleser, R., McMahon, B.T., Shaw, L.R., Marmé, M., and Lam, C.S., An ecological approach to vocational evaluation. In *Work worth doing: Advances in brain injury rehabilitation*. B.T. McMahon and L.R. Shaw (Eds.), Paul M. Deutsch Press, Inc., Orlando, 1991.
3. Cook, J.V. (1990). Returning to work after traumatic head injury. In *Rehabilitation of the adult and child with traumatic brain injury*. M. Rosenthal, E.R. Griffith, M.R. Bond, and J.D. Miller (Eds.), F. A. Davis Company, Philadelphia, (2nd ed.), 1990, 493.

4. Fraser, R.T., Clemmons, D.C., Anderchak, D.A., Dicks, M., and Cook, R. *Vocational re-entry of the traumatic brain injured: A demonstration project.* Paper presented at the National Head Injury Foundation Conference, New Orleans, November, 1990.

5. Wehman, P., Kreutzer, J., West, M., Sherron, P., Zasler, N., Gorah, C., Stonington, H., Burns, C., and Sale, P., Return to work for person with traumatic brain injury: A supported employment approach. *Archives of Physical Medicine and Rehabilitation,* 71, 1042, 1990.

6. Zasler, N.D., The Role of Medical Rehabilitation in Vocational Reentry. *Journal of Head Trauma Rehabilitation.* Aspen Publishers, Inc., 12(5), 42, 1997.

7. Thomas, D.F. and Botterbusch, K.F., The Vocational Assessment Protocol for School-to-Work Transition Programs. *Journal of Head Trauma Rehabilitation.* Aspen Publishers, Inc., 12(2), 48, 1997.

8. Hyler, S.E., Rieder, R.O., Williams, J.B. W., Spitzer, R.L., Hendler, J., and Lyons, M., The Personality Diagnostic Questionnaire: Development and Preliminary Results. *Journal of Personality Disorders,* 2, 229, 1988.

9. Reitan, R.M. and Wolfson, D., *The Halstead-Reitan Neuropsychological Battery.* Neuropsychology Press, Tucson, 1985.

10. Golden, C.J., Hammeke, T., and Purisch, A., *The Luria-Nebraska Battery: Manual* (Rev. Ed.). Western Psychological Services, Los Angeles, 1980.

11. McCarron, L. and Dial, J., *McCarron-Dial Work Evaluation System: Evaluation of the mentally disabled — A systematic approach.* Common Market Press, Dallas, 1976.

12. Acimovic, M.L., Keatley, M.A., and Lemmon, J., The importance of qualitative indicators in the assessment of mild brain injury. *The Journal of Cognitive Rehabilitation,* 8, November/December, 1993.

13. U.S. Department of Labor: *Individual vocational rehabilitation programs: Transition of persons with disability into employment.* Washington, D.C., 1993.

Appendix A

U.S. Department of Labor   Employment Standards Administration
Wage and Hour Division
Washington, D.C. 20210

Statement of principle

The U.S. Department of Labor and community-based rehabilitation organizations are committed to the continued development and implementation of individual vocational rehabilitation programs that will facilitate the transition of persons with disabilities into employment within their communities. This transition must take place under conditions that will not jeopardize the protections afforded by the Fair Labor Standards Act to program participants, employees, employers or other programs providing rehabilitation services to individuals with disabilities.

Guidelines

Where <u>ALL</u> of the following criteria are met, the U.S. Department of Labor will <u>NOT</u> assert an employment relationship for purposes of the Fair Labor Standards Act.

- Participants will be individuals with physical and/or mental disabilities for whom competitive employment at or above the minimum wage level is not immediately obtainable and who, because of their disability, will need intensive ongoing support to perform in a work setting.
- Participation will be for vocational exploration, assessment or training in a community-based placement work site under the general supervision of rehabilitation organization personnel.
- Community-based placements will be clearly defined components of individual rehabilitation programs developed and designed for the benefit of each individual. The statement of needed transition services established for the exploration, assessment or training components will be included in the person's Individualized Written Rehabilitation Plan (IWRP).
- Information contained in the IWRP will not have to be made available, however, documentation as to the individual's enrollment in the community-based placement program will be made available to the Department of Labor. The individual and, when appropriate, the parent or guardian of each individual must be fully informed of the IWRP and the community-based placement component and have indicated voluntary participation with the understanding that participation in such a component does not entitle the participant to wages.

- The activities of the individuals at the community-based placement site do not result in an immediate advantage to the business. The Department of Labor will look at several factors.

    1) There has been no displacement of employees, vacant positions have not been filled, employees have not been relieved of assigned duties, and the individuals are not performing services that, although not ordinarily performed by employees, clearly are of benefit to the business.
    2) The individuals are under continued and direct supervision by either representatives of the rehabilitation facility or by employees of the business.
    3) Such placements are made according to the requirements of the individual's IWRP and not to meet the labor needs of the business.
    4) The periods of time spent by the individuals at any one site or in any clearly distinguishable job classification are specifically limited by the IWRP.

- While the existence of an employment relationship will not be determined exclusively on the basis of the number of hours, as a general rule, each component will not exceed the following limitations:

Vocational explorations	5	hours per job experienced
Vocational assessment	90	hours per job experienced
Vocational training	120	hours per job experienced

- Individuals are not entitled to employment at the business at the conclusion of their IWRP, however, once an individual becomes an employee, the person cannot be considered a trainee at that particular community-based placement unless in a clearly distinguishable occupation.

An employment relationship will exist unless <u>all of the criteria</u> described in the policy are met. If an employment relationship is found to exist, the business will be held responsible for full compliance with the applicable sections of the Fair Labor Standards Act, including those relating to child labor.

Businesses and rehabilitation organizations may, at any time, consider participants to be employees and may structure the program so that the participants are compensated in accordance with the requirements of the Fair Labor Standards Act. Whenever an employment relationship is established, the business may make use of the special minimum wage provisions provided pursuant to section 14(c) of the Act.

Donald J. Hinkel, Chair	Karen R. Keesling, Acting Administrator
National Rehabilitation Facilities	Wage and Hour Division
Coalition	U.S. Department of Labor

Appendix B

Basic vocational evaluation framework

1. *Background information*: Discussion of current medical status, psychosocial history to include family background, available social support, psychiatric/personality difficulties, any substance abuse history), litigation involvement or subsidy claims, and specific financial needs for work entry or re-entry.

2. *Vocational interests*: Summarize results of interest inventories, describe work orientation in relation to Holland codes: Realistic, enterprising, artistic, social, conventional, and investigative whenever appropriate. Discuss need for career exploration, if interests are not well defined.

3. *Review work values or reinforcers* as important to the client.

4. *Neuropsychological results*:
   Assets: Summarize notable to above average capabilities first, then functional abilities that are relatively unimpaired.
   Deficits: Emphasize severe to moderate areas of impairment.
   Emotional/Characterological concerns:

5. *McCarron-Dial Summary*:
   Assets:
   Deficits:

6. *Physical capacities evaluation*:
   The injured worker can:
   Sit for _____ hrs at a time: _____ hrs in an 8-hr day.
   Stand for _____ hrs at a time: _____ hrs in an 8-hr day.
   Walk for _____ hrs at a time: _____ hrs in an 8-hr day.
   Alternately sit/stand for _____ hrs at a time: _____ hrs in an 8-hr day.
   Alternately sit/walk for _____ hrs at a time: _____ hrs in an 8-hr day.
   Alternately stand/walk for _____ hrs at a time: _____ hrs in an 8-hr day.
   Lift (lb capacity) _____freq. _____occas.
   freq. from _____height to _____height.
   Carry _____   freq. _____occas. (_____ x in _____ hrs).
   Push/Pull _____freq. _____occas. (_____ x in _____ hrs).
   _____Squat/Kneel   Frequency:
   _____Bend/Stoop   Frequency:
   _____Crawl   Frequency:
   _____Climb   Ladders/Stairs:

___Reach overhead   Frequency:
___Perform fine manipulation   Yes: No: Comments:
___Operate foot controls   Yes: No:
___Operate hand controls   Yes: No:

7. *Communication*: to include functional academic skill levels:
   a) Ability to follow verbal directions ... How long?
   b) Ability to communicate verbally with public (asking appropriate questions/off topic)?
   c) Follow written directions ... How long?
   d) Ability to use written communication effectively?
   e) Reading level (grade)
   f) Ability to interact appropriately with supervisors (receiving feedback, initiating)?
   g) Ability to sustain attention on a task? Number of minutes:
   h) Ability to show appropriate social demeanor (e.g., no inappropriate laughing, attention-getting gestures, noises, etc.)?

8. *Worker behaviors* (Summary of Worker Performance Assessment or other behaviors observed during testing by other therapists):
   Strengths:
   Concerns:

9. *Summary of work sample performance* (findings from appropriate real work sample, University of Wisconsin-Stout or commercially available sample).

10. *Summary* (includes interests, strengths, areas of deficits/concerns). Specific recommendations relative to:
   a) Specific job goals (identify several viable goals based on synthesized findings and computer search as necessary).
   b) Continuum to placement (will worker need one or more job tryouts/job stations i.e., intermediate evaluation, or can a placement model be chosen–direct placement, on-the-job training, job coach, supervisor or co-worker as mentor, etc.).
   c) Barriers requiring intervention/compensation (i.e., one or more job goals may not be viable without additional rehabilitation engineering or an occupational therapy consult, transportation training, etc.).
   d) Client requires continued vocational exploration or not viable for competitive employment, recommend volunteer or other daily productive activity (discuss specific steps and directions).
   e) This client is not feasible for competitive placement efforts. The focus should be switched to avocational activities and assistance in weekly time structuring).

Reprinted with permission from Robert T. Fraser, Vocational evaluation. *Journal of Head Trauma Rehabilitation*, 1991, 6(3), pp. 52–53.

chapter five

The affirmative industry variation of supported employment

Brian T. McMahon, Ph.D., C.R.C.

Fraser, Clemmons, and McMahon (1990)[1] reported on the utilization of affir-mative industries as a variation on supported employment for adults with severe traumatic brain injury (TBI). An affirmative industry is a nonprofit business entity that provides employment opportunities for adults with severe disabilities that prevent them from competing successfully in the open job market.[2] An affirmative industry has as its primary objective the assertive employment of persons with severe disabilities, as opposed to the production of goods or provision of services for the purpose of generating revenue. Affirmative industries have been developed through hospital outpatient programs. They are particularly helpful to clients in ex-urban or rural post-acute residential TBI rehabilitation facilities, because these communities typ-ically lack a level of commercial activity consistent with the targeted home communities of many clients. Affirmative industries are intended to be used by clients as a transitional, paid evaluation step and a means of vocational exploration. Residential rehabilitation facilities need these programs since they more accurately assess clients' abilities and attempt interventions within actual work sites.

The affirmative industry as supported employment

An affirmative industry can only be distinguished from a sheltered work situation by the way it is designed, structured, operated, and managed. Employees perform real work for real wages, and are typically paid at the minimum wage or higher. Employees are held to performance standards which are as competitive as possible given their current level of vocational functioning. Placement is immediate and precedes the provision of all other support services, and the application of supports is broadened to include job coaching, natural supports, vocational training, job modification, job restructuring, alternative schedules of work, employer education, mentoring, mediation with supervisors, transportation assistance, technical assistance, barrier removal, work adjustment training, on-the-job training, ongoing assessment and re-assessment, and the like. The above are only examples.

The concept of a support is broadened to include any activity which enhances the job maintenance of the individual worker and is bounded only by the creativity limits of the treatment team. These supports are provided as long as is necessary. Work tasks are varied and work settings are integrated.

An affirmative industry which is structured in this way will have face validity for the client, be a normalizing experience, provide focus and meaning for other therapeutic activities, and improve the client's self-perception as a worker. The prevailing management attitude must be that the client will succeed, and individual failures are regarded first as the failures of staff to provide appropriate supports, and not as failures of an uncooperative or incapable client. If planned and developed in this fashion, the affirmative industry can truly be regarded as a variation of supported employment as opposed to sheltered work.

To further distinguish the affirmative industry from a sheltered work experience, clients must be held to realistic hiring and personnel standards. The acquisition of any position in the affirmative industry must conform to normalized protocols, including the procurement of advertised job vacancies, completion of a job application, an employment interview with the hiring manager, and approval of the affirmative industry placement by both the physician and financial sponsor. Failure to acquire written approval from the insuring or financial sponsor, indicating a clear understanding that the affirmative industry is a *rehabilitation* experience and is not to be construed as competitive employment, could jeopardize both the client's benefits and funding for all rehabilitation services. Accordingly, this is a very critical step.

Having accomplished these preliminary steps, a hiring decision is made by a manager. The entire treatment team, with the participation of the client, plans the vocational experience and carefully specifies the nature, scope, and level of appropriate supports. A job offer is extended by the project manager; terms and conditions are negotiated including wages, hours, and start date; W-4, I-9, and other important forms are completed; and the client begins employment with the assistance of supports. During employment in the affirmative industry, the client must be subjected to all the rules of progressive discipline, including verbal and written warnings, reprimand, probation, suspension and termination.

Even with these safeguards, affirmative industries still may be regarded as somewhat more protective than other models of supported employment. It is important to emphasize that affirmative industry arrangements are intended to be short-term, goal-directed, and transitional to more rigorous supported employment options, such as those reviewed by Wehman in Part D. No external recruiting of the client nor long-term planning steps on behalf of the client may occur while the client is involved in the affirmative industry.

Specifics of affirmative industry program development

It is the author's experience that many affirmative industry programs are overplanned, and that this overplanning impedes actual development and may result in abandonment of the entire project. This author began the development of an effective affirmative industry program by accumulating approximately $5,000 through a variety of fundraising activities in the local community. The next steps included securing office space near the residential TBI rehabilitation facility, but far enough away to permit the development of an independent business identity, and incorporating the affirmative industry as a nonprofit, non-tax-exempt business.

The acquisition of freestanding office space in a neighboring commercial district also obviated delays and resistance, which might have occurred in obtaining a zoning variance on the grounds of the facility. Non-tax-exempt status was chosen in the interest of time, because acquiring tax-exempt status would have involved further delays. Moreover, the rehabilitation facility was a proprietary business and it was important to minimize the appearance of any impropriety or conflict of interest in the relationship between the proprietary TBI facility and the nonprofit affirmative industry.

Independent accounting mechanisms, bank accounts, and business operations were established. Equipment, utilities, telephones, and furnishings were procured. The affirmative industry obtained a license as an occupational-leasing company, which gave it the flexibility to offer clients a broad range of work experiences in various integrated community settings, and to provide a valuable resource to community-based employers to meet their needs for temporary labor during peak periods of demand. Fraser et al. (1990)[1] reported a surprising additional benefit of this structure in that several employers who were reluctant to employ certain clients in a supported job arrangement were more open to leasing the same clients from an affirmative industry which absorbed full legal responsibility for the client's productivity, safety, benefits, and insurance. More formal supported employment and other arrangements were later made possible because the affirmative industry, as an employee-leasing company, was able to "broker" the clients' services.

The employee-leasing advantage had the additional benefit of allowing a limited number of more cognitively and behaviorally impaired clients to be leased back to the facility to perform legitimate work on a contractual basis. This minimized the legal, regulatory, and market perception problems which might otherwise be raised in terms of client exploitation. In a number of highly creative instances, the rehabilitation facility was even able to structure the client's treatment regimen as an occupation which the client was "leased" to perform, thus providing tangible reinforcement and at the same time enhancing treatment compliance for some very challenging clients.

In addition, the affirmative industry embarked on a large number of entrepreneurial business ventures on and off the grounds of the facility. Specific legal contracts were arranged for diverse on-grounds activities, which included car washes, greenhouses, woodworking shops, snack bars, canteens, photography services, light auto maintenance, groundskeeping, housekeeping, and others. Clients were very involved in all aspects of the affirmative industry, including project planning and implementation, staffing, accounting, marketing, financial management, and program evaluation. In this way, a large number of occupations were developed over time which were representative of retail sales, service, and light manufacturing industries. Clients were quickly promoted to leadership positions based upon performance, but their tenure therein was brief because these levels of competency, once demonstrated, would trigger the transition to competitive employment or more formal supported jobs arrangements in the community.

It is worth noting that the expeditious development of the affirmative industry only required the redeployment of a single vocational specialist to serve as project manager. Job coaches were recruited directly from the ranks of facility personnel and were assigned to serve the needs of the affirmative industry just as they would any other community employer. It is equally worth noting that by design, job coaches consisted of professional personnel from every discipline, because now these clinicians were permitted and encouraged to perform their therapies within the community, especially in the workplace, whenever possible. The title of job coach was never configured as an independent occupational classification within the company. Therefore, a speech and language pathologist, certified occupational therapy assistant (COTA), vocational rehabilitation counselor, and others were now involved in job coach activities. This is consistent with what has subsequently been termed *disability management* programming, in which therapists perform their duties at the worksite.

In reference to this project, these design features might explain in part what Fraser et al. (1990)[1] observed in the subjective description of successful clients in the affirmative industry. Client initiation, acceptance of verbal instructions, quality and quantity of interaction with supervisors and co-workers, and the willingness to implement treatment strategies in the workplace were observed as characteristics of consistent success, defined as eventual transition to a formal supported or competitive employment setting.

The developers of this program rejected outright the payment of any subminimum wage to affirmative industry employees. Even at minimum wage or higher, many clients with TBI are unrealistic in their vocational expectations — a vocational manifestation of psychological or organically mediated denial. Due to the initial offering of minimum or just above minimum wage jobs, a significant minority of clients at first refused to participate. This level of payment was required to engage most clients, but job development activity on behalf of the clients for more competitive jobs and wages was ongoing. The consistent distribution of weekly paychecks to affirmative industry participants, however, and the fanfare associated with payroll distribution proved to be far more persuasive than the most competent vocational counseling in encouraging resistive clients to participate, if only on an interim basis. Vocational counselors were helpful, however, by emphasizing affirmative industry employment as a routine programming feature, the possibility of rapid advancement, the transitional nature of the program, its value in physical conditioning and cognitive skill improvement, and the proverbial "walk before you run" argument. To maintain credibility, it was imperative that high performers be paid in a manner consistent with their labor market value and transitioned quickly to more competitive environments.

Program benefits

In this program, within three months, work orders for employee leasing and job vacancies to operate the affirmative industry exceeded the number of available clients. Revenues far exceeded the costs of wages, rent, and equipment. After 18 months of operation, program evaluation demonstrated unequivocally that the affirmative industry program extended the reach of employment support to more behaviorally and cognitively impaired TBI clients, and provided an effective bridge to other supported employment placement models. Surprisingly, it was also determined that if affirmative industry participation was the client's only vocational rehabilitation experience, it was as ineffective as no vocational intervention whatsoever. From a company-wide perspective, the percentage of workers' compensation referrals to TBI facilities with an affirmative industry rose by 150% in the first year of operation. The revenues generated from these admissions more than offset any costs to management in terms of program development time and monies.[1]

From a client treatment perspective, the interdisciplinary team was given an abundance of immediate situational assessment data as well as a vocational forum in which to apply their therapies. Clients had access to discretionary monies, which in turn provided independent-living clinicians with a valid basis for budget planning, banking, and the like. Eventual competitive job placement opportunities were maximized because clients were able to provide a record of earnings and a letter of reference from a community employer that was generally not the rehabilitation facility itself.

Administration barriers to affirmative industry implementation

It must be emphasized that facility administrators typically have a range of excuses for delaying or avoiding the development of affirmative industry programs. These include the perception of such programs as sheltered work; the lack of development capital; zoning, licensing, regulatory, or tax-exempt status impediments; the lack of management and clinical and job coaching personnel; the perceived need for subminimum wage certification; and antic- ipated client resistance to lower wages and jobs in the secondary labor market. An intention of this chapter is to emphasize that all of these objec- tions are surmountable. Moreover, there is a genuine need for a variation of supported employment opportunities to be afforded to those TBI clients who are too cognitively or behaviorally involved to participate in more rigorous supported employment models.

An authoritative and helpful resource on the development of affirmative industry programs is given by DuRand (1989).[2] With reference to Minnesota Diversified Industries, DuRand writes extensively on how to define, plan, operationalize, and implement the entrepreneurial concept and apply basic human principles to guide its development and growth. This is a classic reference, which is "must reading" for prospective developers of affirmative industry programs and their perplexed administrators.

Similarly, Barrett and Lavin (1987)[3] have outlined design features of their Industrial Work Model, some of which translate well to the development of an affirmative industry. These include definition, development, marketing, administrative, funding, staffing, and service delivery issues. A myriad of specific examples, protocols, and forms are provided. These developments all grew out of an extensive program evaluation which led to major organi- zational reforms. In this author's opinion, the success of this restructuring is attributable to its adherence to the following philosophical principles.[3]

1. All persons with vocational handicaps are valued individuals no mat- ter how severe their disabilities may be.
2. They deserve the opportunity and choice to work in the least restric- tive, nonsegregated environment possible.
3. They have a right to contribute toward their own self-support and independence.
4. They are capable of acquiring job skills and performing meaningful work in normative business settings when appropriate training and employment support services are available.
5. They deserve to be served by competent staff who are familiar with their disability conditions and capable of producing community em- ployment outcomes.
6. All people will be provided an equal opportunity to work in the open labor market as a first priority regardless of the severity of their disabilities.
7. Our industrial work programs shall be participant-driven to the de- gree possible based on assessed work potential in addition to mar- ketplace opportunities.

8. The high rate of unemployment among person with severe disabilities is a systemic problem which can be resolved by effective leadership, program management, and the application of available training technology and support services.

It is an open management commitment to principles such as these that is the single strongest predictor of success in the development of affirmative industry and related programs.

Both DuRand (1989)[2] and Barrett and Lavin (1987)[3] emphasize the importance of carefully determining the program's definition. Nonetheless, one can overplan such a program and it is helpful to remember that no amount of careful planning or anticipation can prepare staff for the realities of TBI rehabilitative programming. Clients with a TBI and their needs, as professionally assessed, will ultimately guide the development process, while policies and procedures will be frequently and radically amended. Once administration is committed to this direction and appreciates the program benefits, affirmative industry originators will face less resistance, even with required program changes.

Caveats for affirmative industry in the post-ADA era

One of the problems with the early education and implementation of the Americans With Disabilities Act (ADA) of 1990 is the overemphasis on certain illegal forms of discrimination under Title I, the employment provisions. Specifically, far too much is made of failing to provide a reasonable accommodation.

It is worth noting that Title I of the ADA pertains to all aspects of the employment relationship, including recruitment, advertising, job application, hiring, upgrading, promotion, award of tenure, demotion, transfer, layoff, termination, compensation, benefits, training, employer-sponsored activities, and all terms, conditions, or privileges of employment. Furthermore, several other forms of discrimination are expressly outlawed, including "limiting, classifying and segregating" qualified individuals with disabilities. Specifically, Section 102(b)(1) prohibits "...limiting, segregating, or classifying a job applicant or employee because of the disability of such an applicant or employee." This means that many employers (including some who have received recognition and even awards from the rehabilitation community for hiring large numbers of persons with disabilities) might be in violation of the new federal law, if these employees represent similar disabling conditions and/or are segregated in a narrow range of occupations or jobs.

This provision of the law came about because many employers, however benevolent, approached the issue of employing workers with disabilities by asking, "What types of jobs do we have that handicapped people can do?" This is entirely opposite to the spirit of the ADA, which is intended to require careful, case-by-case analysis of each individual applicant or employee, taking into consideration the multipotentiality of each person.

Although it is unclear whether or not affirmative industries are covered entities under the ADA, and it is still somewhat ambiguous how ADA will affect supported employment arrangements, this situation bears monitoring, especially in bench work, mobile work crews, and enclave models of supported employment. As an immediate consideration, the matter of promoting the integration of employees with and without disabilities (which is part of the very definition of supported employment) takes on additional importance in the development of an affirmative industry.

While the regulations to enforce the ADA continue to be refined, there are considerable efforts by all concerned parties to make rigid distinctions between competitive and supported employment. As an example, the Equal Employment Advisory Council (1978),[4] on behalf of employers, is insistent that the provision of a supported employment arrangement is elective and is not required as a reasonable accommodation. True or not, the *supports* developed and demonstrated as effective in supported employment will likely be upheld as examples of reasonable accommodations on a case-by-case basis. Indeed, examples of these include barrier removal; job restructuring; job modification; alternative work schedules; reassignment to a vacant position; modified examinations, training materials, or policies; provision of readers or interpreters; and the provision of specialized equipment or devices. Perhaps the greatest fear for most employers centers around the concept of mandatory "two-for-one" hiring as in the long-term need for interpreters, readers, attendants, or job coaches at the employers' expense.

Under the ADA, an employer may not use a contractual arrangement (such as an employee-leasing agreement with an affirmative industry), which has the effect of subjecting its own qualified applicants or employees with disabilities to discriminatory practices. All of this means that in order to survive in a post-ADA era, affirmative industry will have to represent model human resources practices (in ADA terms), whether or not they are themselves "covered entities" under the law.

References

1. Fraser, R.T., Clemmons, D.C., and McMahon, B.T., Vocational rehabilitation. In J.S. Kreutzer and P.H. Wehman (Eds.) *Community reintegration following traumatic brain injury.* Baltimore: Paul Brookes Publishing Company, 1990, 169.
2. DuRand, J., *Developing an entrepreneurial enterprise.* Menomonie: Materials Development Center, 1989.
3. Barrett, J. and Lavin, D., *The industrial work model: A guide for developing transitional and supported employment.* Menomonie: Materials Development Center, 1987.
4. Equal Employment Advisory Council, Equal employment opportunity for individuals with disabilities. Washington, D.C., 1978.

chapter six

Choice of a placement model

Robert T. Fraser, Ph.D., C.R.C. and Rita Curl, Ph.D.

Introduction

In articles by Fraser (1988),[1] Fraser et al. (1990),[2] and Fraser, Cook, Clemmons, and Curl (1997),[3] a decision-tree framework has been developed to facilitate the choice of a job placement model. This model requires consideration of a number of critical client variables (e.g., neuropsychological, job-related, financial, and emotional/interpersonal) before choosing a placement approach. Figure 1 indicates that despite the level of severity (mild, moderate, severe), the above-referenced client variables are considered in each choice of a placement approach.

In relation to neuropsychological functioning, we are concerned not only with the number of tests outside normal limits and the severity of the impairment, but also the particular pattern of assets and deficits. As discussed by Dr. Uomoto in this text, neuropsychological assets are often not emphasized and they generally need to be considered in placement approaches. The key job-related variables involve the complexity of the work, the amount of time an individual has been involved or trained in a particular job, and the availability/receptivity of the work supervisor or key co-worker to mentoring. Emotional and behavioral issues involve difficulties on the job, which may be caused or exacerbated by the brain injury. The individual's and family's financial need for subsistence must also be considered, within the context of existing subsidies, to include Social Security, and the survivor's capacity to earn money. There are generally specific issues in the above areas which contribute to the choice of placement model. This is not to say that other variables are not considered (e.g., other disabilities, transportation concerns), it is simply that the above variables tend to be standard considerations.

In Figure 1, the reader will note that before the final placement model is chosen, a community job tryout or affirmative industry work activity

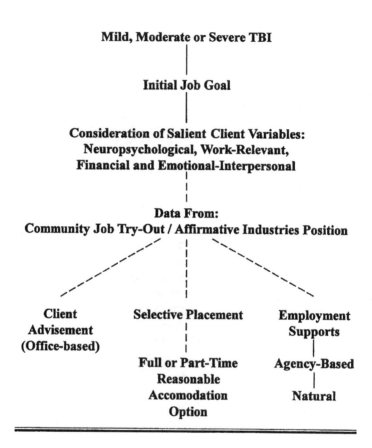

Figure 1   Choosing a Placement Model in Traumatic Brain Injury (TBI).

(which is often involved in an intermediate level of evaluation) may be utilized before the final placement approach is selected. Some of these efforts may be in targeted job areas and result in support of the initial job goal choice. In many cases, however, it is determined that an initial job goal is inappropriate and an alternate goal or goals must be established for a final placement approach. An individual's ability to earn may also result in a modification of the job goal (part-time work so as not to affect an existing subsidy) or establish that a person might do better performing a volunteer activity when productivity is extremely low and cannot be improved with job coaching or assistive technology. With specific vocational goals in mind, a job placement model is ultimately chosen based upon the client variable considerations as previously reviewed. The different models that may be used include the following:

Models

Client advisement or coaching (office-based)

This model is generally used for clients with a mild or moderate range of impairment who are being principally coached to emphasize their residual assets, or in some cases, in the use of specific compensatory strategies to perform adequately and maintain a position. These coached or advisement sessions generally occur in the counselor's or job coach's office. In a number of cases, however, even survivors of a severe injury are still able to profit from this approach. Their ability to use this model will involve the use of more behavioral training (e.g., specific scripts for calling employers) and close monitoring to determine if the approach is feasible and time-efficient.

Using this approach, one client with a mild level of impairment but with visual/spatial memory difficulties, for example, was coached to an on-the-job training situation as a secretary/receptionist because of her difficulties in functioning as a waitress due to a visual/spatial memory deficit. An assistive technology recommendation may still have to be made.

An attorney who had suffered a severe injury was advised to use a 120-item computer software protocol to assist in organizing each case. His organizational abilities were only mildly impaired due to the injury, but his verbal memory deficits were dramatically compromised and the case protocols enabled him to function in a moderately paced legal position within a federal agency.

In general, these clients return to a previous area of work activity, or benefit from short-term vocational counseling and behaviorally oriented job-search skill training. They can make job search errors, etc. but advisement is still a time-efficient and basically effective approach. They have enough residual cognitive abilities to, in fact, call in for compensatory strategy recommendations if they encounter difficulties in job search activity.

Selective placement

This type of model involves direct placement activity or brokering on behalf of a client for whom a job match is based upon some of the key client-related variables as previously reviewed. Following the placement or brokering activity, interaction or intervention with the employer tends to be minimal. Follow-up with the employer, unless difficulties are obvious, tends to be at established monitoring points (e.g., 15, 30, 60, 90, and 180 days). It may be necessary, if the client is being trained on the job through an on-the-job-training contract mechanism, to monitor the situation more closely, to ensure that the training is occurring and being absorbed by the trainee. In general, however, for this type of approach, it is assumed that ongoing support within the workplace is not necessary. This is not to say, however, that some type of reasonable accommodation (viz., procedural, physical modification to the work site, or assistive technology may have to be considered — see Warren, Chapter three of this text).

Ongoing contact with the client and/or significant others may be maintained more closely than with the employer. Some clients are placed on a part-time basis largely due to the effects of the injury on their cognitive and physical functioning and a reduced capacity to earn money. Full-time work may also affect their financial subsidies so drastically that a person's or family's basic economic well-being is at risk. As an example, what they are capable of earning on a full-time basis may be dramatically less than their Social Security income. (Note: Work-related expenses may need to be evaluated in order to use one of the mechanisms available for maintenance of Social Security benefits.)

Forms of employment support

Employment support can be categorized under two categories: (a) supports that are directly provided by a rehabilitation *agency* or organization; and (b) supports that are more naturally provided by private sector companies at the job site.

Agency-based supports

Employment-related supports that can be consistently attributed to the rehabilitation agency include the following:

Community training consultant

One job placement option is for the rehabilitation agency or organization to hire a community training consultant to take responsibility for both the training and placement of the traumatically brain-injured client. Within a funded NIDRR demonstration project,[2] a sub-group of clients with severe traumatic brain injuries required intensive training which could not be accommodated completely within a formal classroom situation or through the use of a job coach. Examples of trainers receiving contracts for individualized training included a community college teacher (e.g., a welder) and a retired community professional (e.g., a pharmacist). The welding instructor had a client as a student within the formal classroom (lab) situation, but worked with him for an additional one and a half hours a day after the formal class, and assumed responsibility for the client's job placement. The instructor was paid directly by the state vocational rehabilitation agency. In another instance, a retired pharmacist worked with a client within a mail-order pharmaceutical company until appropriate productivity and accuracy criteria were achieved. In some instances, this consultant activity will be accomplished on a paid contractual basis with the rehabilitation agency, but in other instances by a committed community volunteer (e.g., a retired professional).

Job sharing, contractual arrangement

Sowers (1989)[4] has described a number of examples of a support co-worker model being used with a job that is actually shared by persons with and without a disability. In these cases, the rehabilitation agency is paid for a specified amount of work (e.g., making a certain number of deli meals daily) for which it subsequently hires a nondisabled worker and a client with a disability to complete the work activity. The worker without a disability is paid a specified amount and the worker with a disability may be paid based upon productivity or an established wage. This arrangement becomes very feasible through contractual monies received from the involved company, state rehabilitation agency training funds, or other merged funds (e.g., supported employment monies). The Sowers Oregon program had teams involved in contracted photocopying work, sandwich delivery, drapery dry-cleaning, legal office tasks, and item unpacking and pricing. In utilizing this approach, the agency identifies jobs or job tasks that a person with a TBI would be able to perform independently or with minimal ongoing support within the required work tasks.

Supported employment

Presently there are a number of models of supported employment that are used nationally. The *enclave* model involves a small group of workers (usually four to eight) who receive long-term training and supervision at a host company. In some instances they are working together (e.g., around a specific assembly task), but in other cases they may be conducting diverse tasks within a restaurant, hotel, or mail-order company and receiving intermittent supervision. Another well-established model is the *mobile work crew*. This type of crew involves four to six individuals working with a supervisor, and all workers being paid by a specific nonprofit organization. As indicated by Wehman (1990, p. 189),[5] this type of model is very viable in rural areas in which the needs of the community can be identified and met over an expanded geographical area. The *entrepreneurial or small business option* is another supported employment model in which a small group of workers with disabilities is paired with a supervisor without a disability and/or co-workers in one specific small business such as printing, snowmobile servicing, a flower shop, or a mail-order operation.

In traumatic brain injury rehabilitation, the individual supported employment model as popularized by Dr. Paul Wehman and colleagues at the Medical College of Virginia, may be appropriate most often. This can be the case particularly when individuals have specific or specialized prior work backgrounds which can be utilized in work entry or re-entry. It involves a one-to-one job coach-to-client support ratio. Approaches are individualized for the job placement, training, and stabilization needs of the client with TBI. In Chapter seven, Dr. Wehman reviews the approach that was taken in a study sponsored by the National Institute on Disability and Rehabilitation Research (NIDRR) in which 77% of 59 clients were placed in competitive jobs.[6] Following this study, Dr. Wehman's staff have provided ongoing vocational services to survivors with a TBI and continue to clarify outcomes using the individualized job-coach model.[7]

Natural supports in the workplace

Supports that are more consistently provided through a company within the work setting include the following:

Employer or supervisor as training mentor

For a number of individuals with severe cognitive difficulties, the immediate employer or supervisor will be the best training option. This is true for a number of reasons. In some cases, the job is simply too complex or specialized and a job coach would not have the aptitude or would require an extended learning period to grasp even the basic rudiments of the job. Some companies simply prefer to use their own personnel for training. Other companies are committed to Affirmative Action hiring, but still do not wish to have non-company personnel on the premises. A particular benefit of this approach is that the supervisor/employer feels empowered not only to train, but to handle additional difficulties when they arise on the job. This is not to say that a job coach or rehabilitation counselor may not be involved in the initial framing of the training, assisting with a behavioral management plan, or be available for troubleshooting, etc.; it simply means that the primary responsibility is assumed by the supervisor or employer. On-the-job training funds are often used as a means of compensating the employer or supervisor for the training time. It may be helpful for both the individual and supervisor or co-worker to understand that the company is being financially compensated for this effort and further establish commitment to the training endeavor. These on-the-job training agreements are frequently developed for periods of up to three months and sometimes longer, using state rehabilitation agency funds, special Department of Labor[8] funding, etc.

Co-worker assistance

Although a relatively new job placement model in traumatic brain injury vocational rehabilitation, this approach appears to have considerable potential. The potential co-worker roles include those of trainer, observer, and advocate for the client within the workplace. A large part of the advocacy for clients with traumatic brain injury may involve the education of co-workers and other staff about a client's specific cognitive assets and deficits. In this manner, the new worker is not simply categorized as a person with a "brain injury," but a person with a specific type of deficit (e.g., a spatial memory difficulty). Co-workers who understand the individual's "nonvisible" deficits are more likely to be cooperative and to support the client.

Shafer, Tait, Keen and Jesiolowski (1989)[9] reviewed the growing literature regarding the involvement of co-workers in the supported employment process. Additionally, they present a number of case studies in which co-workers are primarily involved in providing consumers with specific forms of performance-based feedback on the specific job data collected. Shafer et al. underscore that the benefits of this approach are that employee performance data are more likely to be reliable and provide a realistic perspective on employment performance. Second, they emphasize that there is a greater potential that the data will capture the necessary, but often subtle performance standards within the industry. A final advantage is that a performance-based feedback structure gives a co-worker a framework for feedback and may remind a co-worker to, in fact, provide this important information.

A perspective on co-worker and employer training programs

Although still being refined, it is important to review some of the available information on the training of co-workers to engage in the job training and maintenance functions. Work by Sowers and Powers (1989)[4] and Fraser et al. (1990)[2] suggested that this is an area that demands further exploration of program implementation with the survivor of a TBI. One of the most convincing arguments is that in a study by Fraser, Dikmen, McLean, and Temkin (1988)[10] 92% of those working at the time of injury were involved in semi-skilled or skilled jobs at the time of injury. In preparation for returning them to the workplace, there will simply be an inadequate number of skilled job coaches who can assist in retraining or otherwise stabilizing them within their prior jobs. Job coaches or transition specialists will often be needed to frame the training paradigm, be involved in some of the initial acquisition training, intervene in crises, etc. There is no question, however, that when difficulties tend to involve more job-specific complex skill training and skill generalization or maintenance, co-worker involvement will be critical, particularly for those in skilled occupations.

Implementing a co-worker training program

For purposes of actually implementing a program of this nature, the reader is referred to manuals created at the Developmental Center for Handicapped Persons at Utah State University, Logan, Utah. Dr. Rita Curl and colleagues developed both manuals and a video series that were initially provided for use with workers with developmental disabilities, but have great applicability for the population with TBI. The materials go beyond the role of the co-worker as an observer/data collector or advocate, but actually emphasize in detail the training function. The manuals *Put That Person to Work!: A Manual for Implementors using the Co-worker Training Model,*[11] and *Put That Person to Work!: A Co-Worker Training Manual for the Co-Worker Transition Model,*[12] are for agency personnel who are attempting to implement this co-worker training model. Highlights from these works include the following:

Identification of co-workers as trainers

- They should be above average or "master" workers who are well liked by peers and management.
- They must make a commitment to learn to train, observe and collect data, and employ advocacy strategies.
- They need to understand the client's assets and deficits to effectively advocate for him or her within the workplace.

Commitment of management and supervisors
Management must agree to some of the following:

- Training periods for employees with a TBI will routinely be longer than for those without disabilities.
- Co-workers will have training responsibilities and will need to have an appropriate work schedule.
- Co-worker recording of training performance data and periodic visits from rehabilitation agency personnel need to be accepted and supported.
- Financial arrangements with the company for co-worker payment, on-the-job training funds, etc. also must be clearly understood. In most cases, the co-worker is paid directly by hour or segments of an hour (e.g., during lunch, while on break, etc.) while training the client. A recent example was an architect paid $24 an hour (his hourly fee) to train a client between 4:30 and 5:30 p.m. at the end of the work day. Another mechanism could involve paying a co-worker an additional two dollars an hour, or through increasing percentages of co-worker salaries for the additional training help they provide. At certain junctures, the co-worker training or coaching time becomes minimal, but the activity occurs on company time. In several instances, we determined what these accumulated minutes cost the company over several months and simply reimbursed the company for the co-worker's time with the trainee. This might only involve two or three hundred dollars over several months, but the reimbursement seems appreciated — especially by small companies. Funding for the co-worker's salary or payments can come from a state vocational rehabilitation agency, on-the-job training contracts, Department of Labor[8] demonstration grants, monies designated for that purpose through a Social Security PASS or IWRE Plan, etc., or directly from a committed company.
- Management must commit to providing support when the designated training co-worker is not at work and make use of available support from transition specialists.
- There should be a commitment to conduct additional client training before/after work or on breaks, as necessary.

Training

- Co-workers are taught to follow the tell, show, watch, and coach teaching sequence as outlined in the manual by Curl et al. (1987).[11]
- Following in-service training, rehabilitation counselors or job coaches participate in job training with co-workers and trainees to identify the accuracy with which co-workers implement strategies presented in the manuals and videotapes. Trainer-implemented tools (e.g., tape-recorded sessions, one-minute reminders, bonus and warning systems, work set-up recommendations, picture checklists, timers, or self-evaluation strategies) may be needed when trainees demonstrate performance deficits.
- Job coach or rehabilitation personnel may visit, initially as often as daily, to assess the acceptability of a trainee's job skills by reviewing the performance checklist completed by a co-worker or supervisor. Additional co-worker assistance may be provided as necessary. With job coach or rehabilitation counselor input, decision-tree information is available from the co-worker training manual relative to different trainer-implemented tools that can be used for specific areas of encountered difficulties[11] — (see Figure 2).
- There must be a commitment to ongoing support of the trainee, not only to document performance, but to assess co-worker and supervisor satisfaction for guiding future interventions and document overall program effectiveness. Checklist evaluations involve the co-worker's or supervisor's recording of time and accuracy data, while performance questionnaires are used to assess how well the trainee is doing in the eyes of his or her co-workers and supervisors. Copies of all these forms are provided in the manual by Curl and Hall (1990, Appendix D).[12]

Ongoing support of the co-worker program

- Adequate time must be budgeted for job coach, co-worker, and client to engage in the training process.
- The psychological fitness of the job coach and rehabilitative counseling staff must be promoted to effectively work with the diverse needs of the employment community and the agency's clients in training.
- Job coaches and rehabilitation counselors must be responsible only for decisions in which they have the academic, employment-related, or additional required expertise. Additionally, co-worker trainers should be discouraged from independently choosing a training intervention or a training tool (e.g., bonus/warning, timer, self-evaluation). They should not be given the responsibility of resolving performance or interpersonal difficulties without the guidance of the rehabilitation counselor or job coach. Outside consultation for the job

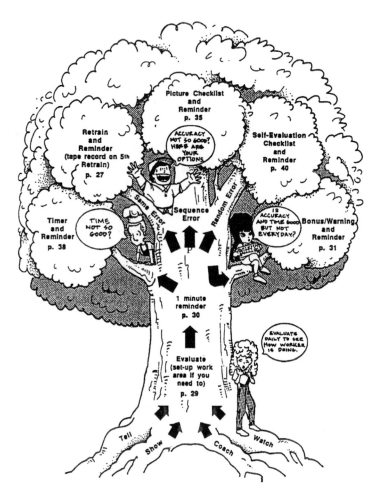

Figure 2   Intervention decision tree.

coach or rehabilitation counselor should be available as necessary from a behavioral psychologist or special educator.

Program monitoring
- Supervision at all levels is responsible for monitoring to ensure that services are provided according to the specifications of the service agency.

In co-worker training, it would appear that much of the procedures used by job coach or supported employment specialists parallel those described by Dr. Wehman in the next chapter. Key differences will involve the ongoing tutoring received by co-worker trainers relative to training strategies and the compensatory measures utilized. An experienced job coach will be operating at a more sophisticated level as a "trainer to these co-worker trainers." Although job coaches often use co-workers as training aids, the work by Curl and colleagues provides discrete procedures and monetarily compensates employees for their commitment instead of more informal or casual arrangements.

Benefits to the co-worker as trainer model in providing natural support

Although natural supports have increasingly been discussed in the literature,[13] Dr. Curl and colleagues have provided the field of rehabilitation with discrete procedures outlined in manuals and videotapes. As previously discussed, Figure 2 presents the intervention decision tree as offered in the manual[11] for intervening with an individual experiencing cognitive difficulties at the work site. Above the basic training procedure, this type of framework is very helpful for the co-worker trainer. At times, however, the co-worker trainer will still need input from an employment specialist, rehabilitation counselor, or even a behavioral psychologist/special educator working as a consultant.

Some common types of interventions for employees with traumatic brain injuries include small dictation aids used to *remember*, particularly extraneous details or details without a specific context. Sequenced tasks lists can be important even for individuals performing relatively complex work activity (e.g., installing showers or kitchen floors). Due to attentional deficits or tendencies to get tangential in work activities, timed work segments can be very helpful. With timelines linked to work activity, it is very common for productivity to increase dramatically and disinhibited behavior or random tangential activity to decrease substantially. In the case of an architect who was excessively talkative and verbally disinhibited on the job site, simple time deadlines for segments of architectural plans increased productivity from 25 to 50%, while virtually eliminating random verbal intrusions into the conversations of others.

A number of working survivors also respond well to bonus and warning systems. Some of these approaches may be a little more sophisticated than those used with groups having developmental disabilities. For example, a supervisor gave one survivor with a rather aggrandized self-perception, 30 minutes at the end of the work week for area phone contacts and "political networking" after his basic job duties as a custodial work services liaison to area businesses was completed in a timely and business-like fashion. Time involved in this type of phone activity was highly reinforcing to this survivor. He viewed himself as politically tied into activities within the city. This "time-to-make contacts" reinforcer further assisted in keeping him at his work tasks during the week and was basically harmless.

It should be noted that at times material from the manual might be abstracted for the co-worker trainer because the present format may appear to "talk down" to the co-worker trainer involved in skilled or professional work. Nevertheless, the system is based upon well-developed behavioral principles and has very practical value in most instances of job-site performance deficit or adjustment concerns.

Findings from a co-worker as trainer project in TBI vocational rehabilitation

A three-year study was undertaken by Drs. Fraser, Curl, Clemmons, and colleagues involving the provision of service to 120 clients with severe traumatic brain injury between October 1993 through September 1996 in urban Seattle, Washington and at a rural site in Minot, North Dakota.* The thrust of the study was to determine the effectiveness of applying Dr. Curl's co-worker trainer model to the TBI population. In general, participants approximated 34 years of age, averaged 17 days in coma, 90% were male, and they approximated 13 years of education.[3] The group also averaged about nine years from injury with slightly more than half being supported on Social Security or another form of subsidy. Although neuropsychological testing indicated an overall moderate degree of impairment, deficits were most evident on tests tapping cognitive flexibility and speed of information processing (e.g., Trails B or the Wechsler - R Digit Symbol subtest).

A procedural overview of the project included the following sequence of steps: a) standardized review of existing client medical, psychosocial, and psychological information followed by a comprehensive intake session or sessions; b) neuropsychological assessment; c) vocational evaluation and goal setting; d) the use of a two- to three-month short-term work trial(s) or community job tryout(s); e) the use of a weekly psychoeducational group that reviewed adjustment issues and promoted specific psychosocial skill building (e.g., conversational skills); and f) review of each client's salient variables in choosing a vocational placement model as in the Figure 1 Placement Decision Tree.

It is of interest that even within a group experiencing severe TBI, there is a considerable amount of functional heterogeneity. Based upon early intake and assessment information, it is often difficult to determine whether an individual might profit from a co-worker as trainer model, or the appropriateness of any specific job placement model. This can require both time and situational assessment.

Of 88 individuals referred to the Seattle project (more follow-up data were available at the urban site), 51 secured longer-term employment lasting more than two months, 14 secured employment lasting two months, with four achieving only very short-term employment. Individuals *who utilized*

* This research was partially funded by Grant No. H-128A 30040-95 from the U.S. Department of Eduation Office of Special Education and Rehabilitation Services.

only one placement model could be grouped as follows: self-referred to a job (n = 9), requiring vocational counseling assistance only (n = 13), requiring selective placement or brokering to an employer (n = 14), requiring co-worker as trainer support (n = 15), or requiring job coaching (n = 3). In a number of other instances, it was helpful to match models, e.g., two weeks of job coaching transitioning to a formal co-worker as trainer placement model. It is often the situational assessment at an intermediate level of vocational evaluation that establishes the model to be used and/or the need for a blended model.

Further review of findings from the Co-Worker Project at the Seattle site suggested that at a 14-month follow-up, despite the model utilized, all placed participants from the program were working 75–85% of the time vs. about one-third of the time pre-involvement with the program.[3] All of those placed improved dramatically from pre-project status. There is *no approach that is necessarily better than another* — the perspective is really, "What is most appropriate for each individual?" Earnings varied from $6.53 to $8.34 an hour by model group, but this again does not argue for the effectiveness of one approach vs. another. As an example, those using co-workers were often trying to return to more complex jobs that they'd held before — the nature of the job dictating a higher salary structure. Some individuals who could be counseled from the office relative to their job search were simply less cognitively impaired and didn't need a placement approach with more support.

For the co-worker model "per se," there are again a number of obvious *benefits*:

a) supervisors feel empowered to handle situation; b) interactive relationships are built for the client; c) co-workers are available and provide ongoing strategies; and d) for skilled and semi-skilled positions, this may be the approach of necessity. Preliminary findings also indicate cost efficiency, within a range of $100–$400 per co-worker payments at more than one year on the job for the client. The Seattle clients were again a group with severe TBI. Those being trained by a co-worker averaged 17 days spent in coma. This appears to be extremely cost-efficient as compared with other forms of supported employment. Wehman et al.[7] report job coach, supported employment with cost ranges of $6,000 to $12,000. Even with supportive agency counseling, placement, and set-up costs for the model within the $2,000 range, the co-worker as trainer model appears to be an efficient option.

Findings from the co-worker model, however, remain preliminary as applied to the population with a traumatic brain injury. The above data are only from the one demonstration project. Training requirements can often be too overwhelming for a co-worker trainer and an employment specialist will need to be brought in from the agency. Case management concerns (e.g., transportation or medical concerns) can also demand an employment specialist. Some clients will not want a co-worker to understand their cognitive limitations, certain companies won't commit to the model or might change their training commitment during business peaks, etc. Nevertheless, it shows considerable promise as a rehabilitation placement tool, especially for those entering semi-skilled to skilled work.

Summary

This section has reviewed the major placement options: client advisement or coaching (office-based), selective placement (full- and part-time), and forms of employment support. Forms of support are further categorized into agency-based supports (community training consultant, job-sharing contractual work, and supported employment) and natural supports (supervisor/employer or co-workers as trainers). Additional reviews of issues related to the co-worker as trainer were provided because this remains a relatively formative model for the population with traumatic brain injury. Considering, however, the skilled work background of many TBI survivors, it is a logical area for refinement as a placement approach. It is an approach that can be used by itself or paired with another support model.

References

1. Fraser, R.T., Refinement of a decision tree in traumatic brain injury job placement. *Journal of Rehabilitation Education*, 6, 179, 1988.
2. Fraser, R.T., Clemmons, D.C., and McMahon, B.T., Vocational rehabilitation. In J.S. Kreutzer and P.H. Wehman (Eds.), *Community reintegration following traumatic brain injury.* Baltimore: Paul Brookes Publishing Company, Baltimore, 1990, 169.
3. Fraser, R.T., Cook, R., Clemmons, D.C., and Curl, R.H., Work access in traumatic brain injury rehabilitation. *Physical Medicine and Rehabilitation Clinics of North America.* Vol. 8(2), 371, 1997.
4. Sowers, J., Supported employment models and approaches for persons with physical and multiple disabilities. In J. Sowers and L. Powers (Eds.), *Vocational preparation and employment of students with physical and multiple disabilities.* Oregon Research Institute, Portland, 1989.
5. Wehman, P., Support employment: Model implementation and evaluation. In J.S. Kreutzer and P.H. Wehman (Eds.), *Community reintegration following traumatic brain injury.* Paul Brookes Publishing Company, Baltimore, 1990, 185.
6. Wehman, P., Kreutzer, J., West, M., Sherron, P., Zasler, N., Gorah, C., Stonington, H., Burns, C., and Sale, P., Return to work for persons with traumatic brain injury: A supported employment approach. *Archives of Physical Medicine and Rehabilitation*, 71, 1042, 1990.
7. Wehman, P.H., West, M.D., Kregel, J., et al. Return to work for persons with severe traumatic brain injury: A data-based approach to program development, *Journal of Head Trauma Rehabilitation*. 10, 27, 1995.
8. U.S. Department of Labor. Individual vocational rehabilitation programs: *Transition of persons with disability into employment.* Washington, D.C., (1993).
9. Shafer, M., Tait, K., Keen, R., and Jesiolowski, C., Supported competitive employment: Using co-workers to assist follow-along efforts. *Journal of Rehabilitation*, Apr.-Jun., 68, 1989.

10. Fraser, R.T., Dikmen, S., McLean, A., and Temkin, N., *Employability of head injured survivors: The first year post-injury.* Rehabilitation Counseling Bulletin, 31, 278, 1988.
11. Curl, R.M., McConaughy, E.K., Pawley, J.M., and Salzberg, C.L., *Put that person to work!: A co-worker training manual for the co-worker transition model.* Outreach, Development and Dissemination Division, Developmental Center for Handicapped Persons, Utah State University, Logan, 1987.
12. Curl, R.M. and Hall, S.M., *Put that person to work!: A manual for implementors using the co-worker training model.* Outreach, Development, and Dissemination Division, Developmental Center for Handicapped Persons, Utah State University, Logan, 1990.
13. Storey, K. and Certo, N.J., *Natural supports for increasing integration in the work place for people with disabilities: A review of the literature and guidelines for implementation.* Rehabilitation Counsel Bulletin, 40, 62, 1996.

chapter seven

Supported employment for persons with traumatic brain injury: a guide for implementation

Paul Wehman, Ph.D., John Bricout, Ph.D., and Pam Targett, M.Ed.

Introduction

Individuals with traumatic brain injury who would like to work often face formidable challenges. Severe injury can result in deficits in cognition, memory, mobility, physical ability, and psychosocial functioning that deter employment.

Cognitive issues in areas of slow speed of information processing, decrease in the ability to attend and concentrate, and impaired memory affect the ability to learn and/or perform tasks. Another issue is change in executive functioning which compromises the person's ability to organize, prioritize, and carry out functions.[1-3] These are important attributes for learning and performing work tasks in most businesses.

Traumatic brain injury seldom occurs isolated from physical injury to a sensory or motor system. Severe physical limitations, lack of coordination, and motor slowness can adversely restrict the person's capacity for return to a former job as well as limit the range of future work opportunities.[4,5]

Several authors have cited diminished social functioning including lowered frustration tolerance level, depression, and an inability to demonstrate acceptable social etiquette as major barriers to successful vocational outcomes for people who sustain TBI.[6,7] Sometimes individuals will experience a reduced capacity to get along with others, or difficulties with impulsiveness or controlling frustration. An inability to acknowledge social cues can also lead to difficulties for the person.[8]

Individuals are also likely to encounter environmental and transportation barriers, limited or antiquated vocational assistance, and social isolation.[9] There is no doubt that persons who sustain TBI experience difficulties that lead to serious obstacles to employment.

Faced with an array of complex issues, it comes as no surprise that studies investigating employment outcomes following traumatic brain injury have not been encouraging. Post-injury employment rates have ranged from twenty-two to fifty-five%.[4,10,11,12] Furthermore, high unemployment rates persist at long intervals of seven to fifteen years after injury.[4,6,11]

To effectively address the vocational futures of survivors with TBI, many professionals have called for more proactive and holistic programs. Supported employment offers such an approach. Inherent to the success of supported employment is the availability of long-term supports that are readily available and can be accessed by the individual being served, the customer, with ease. Such programs are dedicated to assisting people with severe disabilities with going to work and providing select case management services. Case management focuses on initially alleviating existing problems and proactively planning ways to reduce the occurrence of future ones.

Only in recent years has supported employment been viewed as a viable alternative for individuals with severe traumatic brain injury. Outcome reports have tended to be favorable; participants greatly increased their earnings to approximately their pre-injury levels.[13,14] Results also indicate that while receiving services, individuals were employed an average of two-thirds of their total service time.[15] This finding also reveals that some individuals experience frequent job changes either due to the problems they exhibit or their need to relearn job preferences and/or work skills. Fortunately, job tenure tends to improve over time.[5]

Initiating and maintaining a supported employment program: description of supported employment

Supported Employment evolved from research and demonstration projects in the late 1970s and early 1980s which showed that persons with severe physical, cognitive, and behavioral disabilities who were historically relegated to work shops or deemed "inappropriate" for vocational rehabilitation (VR) services, could work in the community if afforded the opportunity and support. Unlike traditional vocational rehabilitation models which initially focused on "curing," "fixing," or "prevocationally training" individuals with significant disabilities, supported employment promotes individualized supports in natural work environments. This concept of supporting individuals has been extended to education, housing, recreation, family assistance, and other areas.

The reason for development of this model was to meet the particularly challenging vocational needs of people with very severe disabilities. Supported employment has been used very successfully, for example, with individuals with moderate, severe, and profound mental retardation and significant physical disabilities who did not benefit from the traditional placement approaches of vocational rehabilitation.

Supported employment became a service option within the VR service system through the Rehabilitation Act Amendments of 1986. The Act made supported employment a viable option in all fifty states under the Title 6C program. There are also ample discretionary funding opportunities to initiate supported employment programs for people with severe disabilities, including those with TBI.

Two changes in the Rehabilitation Act Amendments of 1992 have had significant effects on the design and delivery of supported employment. First, the increasing use of natural supports within supported employment implementation and second, increasing control over vocational goals and service delivery to the customer with a disability.

Natural supports

West (1996)[9] states that natural supports is a term used to refer to the informal support networks that all persons develop to enhance happiness and functional performance in our communities and workplaces. Natural supports should be utilized in employment services for individuals with disabilities. Employee assistance programs, public accommodations, such as transportation services, community service organizations, and assistance provided by worksite personnel are natural supports.[16,17]

Natural supports have particular significance for persons with severe brain injuries who are in need of supported employment services. The supported employment regulations require that sources to pay for and provide ongoing support be available, or that there is reason to believe they will be available, prior to the initiation of services. In many states, persons who acquire brain injuries as adults do not have ready access to extended-service funding streams, which are usually marked for individuals with mental retardation and developmental disability, particularly if the injury occurred after the age of 11.[18] Planning for natural supports (e.g., a co-worker as trainer) as the extended service option can make supported employment available to individuals with brain injuries who might otherwise not be able to access services due to the absence or uncertainty of a readily available extended funding source.

West (1995)[19] also reports that the availability of natural support at the work site can have very positive impacts on employment outcomes. A study of 37 individuals with severe brain injuries who were placed into supported employment positions concluded that the social support and economic aspects of a position are two very important but often overlooked factors in promoting return to work among survivors.

Self-determination and choice

The Rehabilitation Act Amendments of 1992 signaled a new era in disability services in America. The Act explicitly states that disability does not diminish the right of individuals to experience self-determination and to make informed choices. Furthermore, it requires services to promote choice and self-determination.

The new choice amendments to the Rehabilitation Act allow VR consumers to have control over decisions regarding career and job goals services, service providers, and methods.[9] With these changes, the role of vocational rehabilitation agencies shifts from a gatekeeper of services and funds to the purchase of services as a customer service organization where the client is considered the key arbiter of appropriate goals and services.[19] This new paradigm has been given such names as consumer-initiated, customer-directed, or customer-focused services.

Wehman et al. (1995)[15] described a customer-initiated supported employment program that promotes and maximizes the participation of the person with the disability. Forty-eight individuals, the majority of survivors of TBI, went to work and 52% remained employed when the demonstration project ended. On average, participants worked 25 hours per week, earned $4.89 per hour, and accumulated $687.00 in wages per month. Among those who stopped work, approximately 17% were terminated by their employer. Reasons included poor attendance, inability to work hours needed, and inappropriate behaviors.

Description of supported employment models

From its inception, supported employment has been characterized by individual or group option arrangements. First, there is the individual placement model which utilizes a single staff person, an employment specialist who provides support to the person with help locating work and directly on the job-site when the individual becomes employed. The employment specialist provides intervention on the job until the new employee becomes increasingly able to fulfill all performance expectations. As the employee gains competency, the employment specialist fades his or her presence from the site. However, the employment specialist continues to visit the employee at work and provides support either on or off the worksite as needed.

There are also three types of group models as previously discussed. One is commonly referred to as the *industrial enclave*, a second the *mobile work crew*, and a third the *small business model*. The group options are mentioned here for informational purposes only. The authors of this book do not advocate the use of this approach for people with traumatic brain injuries. It is important to note that over the years there has been a sharp decline in the number of people participating in group options and significant growth in the individual placement model. What follows in the section below is a more detailed description of each of the models.

Individual placement model

The individual placement model is an employment approach for individuals with moderate and severe disabilities which enables them to become employed in the typical labor market for wages commensurate with the pay of other workers. In this approach, an employment specialist provides individualized assistance and support that enables the person to consider career options, locate work, access accommodations including individualized job skills training at the workplace, and receive ongoing support.[20] When a potential job is identified, the employment specialist analyzes the work tasks and environment and then counsels the customer on how the opportunity meets his preferences and capitalizes on the person's abilities. Potential support needs are also identified and discussed. Once the person is hired, the employment specialist either assists with accessing supports and/or provides service as needed. As the new employee gains the necessary skills to work independently and performance reaches the employer's standards, the employment specialist gradually reduces the time and intensity of support. The employment specialist may provide additional training, advocacy, and support whenever necessary. For example, additional training on the job may be warranted if there has been a change of job duties or how the work is done, or if a new supervisor is hired. Other factors that may indirectly or directly adversely affect the employee's work stability may also prompt attention from the employment specialist.

Benefits of the individual placement model

1. Gives customers choice in selecting work opportunities that meet their individual preferences and abilities. Career opportunities are only limited by what the community has to offer.
2. Offers the greatest opportunity for integration among non-disabled workers and the general public, since work takes place in typical jobs.
3. Does not group the individual with the disability with other individuals with disabilities since it may diminish self-confidence and increase inappropriate behaviors.
4. Allows the individual to earn competitive wages[21] and receive benefits.
5. Allows the customer to participate in the employment process to the fullest extent made possible by individual abilities.

Mobile work crews

The mobile work crew model of supported employment consists of a number of workers with severe disabilities (generally four to eight) and one supervisor, who is usually a human-service worker with a supported employment agency. The crew typically travels from one business to another, performing custodial work, grounds maintenance, housecleaning, janitorial, and other needed services in the community. Work contracts are drawn up between the different agencies and the human-service worker provides the training, supervision, and transportation from site to site, and never leaves the job-site. Potential for contact with the general public is an important consideration in work site selection to ensure optimal integration opportunities. Integration usually takes place when the crew interacts with the general public during breaks and lunchtime. This model is flexible to the local job market and is able to meet the needs of urban, suburban, or rural areas.[22-24]

Enclaves in industry

The enclave is one of the most commonly accepted supported employment models. It is characterized by a group (generally five to eight) or fewer workers with severe disabilities who are trained and supervised by a human-service worker within a local business. The individuals are employed in an integrated host business or industry and access employment opportunities provided to all employees of the host business or industry. Enclaves pay wages commensurate to the individual's productivity and may be paid directly by the host business or industry or the human-services support organization.[16] The human-service worker does not fade from the job-site. The ability to provide continuous supervision and flexible and shared decision making between the host business or industry and the human-service support organization is one of the advantages of the enclave model.[22]

Entrepreneurial model

The entrepreneurial model is a manufacturing or subcontract not-for-profit operation employing approximately 15 individuals with severe disabilities, as well as workers without disabilities, and providing one type of product or service. Typically, the individuals with severe disabilities have spent most of their lives in institutions and often display inappropriate social behaviors, making it difficult for them to be accepted in competitive employment environments. This supported employment option was developed by Specialized Training Program (STP) at the University of Oregon.

The individuals with severe disabilities are trained and supervised by two to three human-service workers who do not leave the job-site. The model relies on contractual assembly work;[26] therefore, the success of the program depends on securing ongoing contract work from industry. Workers are generally paid sub-minimum wages commensurate to their productivity.[27] Typically, companies using this model share the profits among all employees through salary increases, bonuses, improved benefits, and profit sharing. Management salaries are usually funded through local agencies as monitored by a board of directors.

Persons should be considered as potential candidates for group model options only when multiple repeated attempts at the individual approach have not lead to increased success or if someone expresses a desire for this type of option. Anyone who ever becomes involved in a group employment option should be routinely assessed for their potential to engage in an individualized career search.

All research resulting from the Supported Employment Program at Virginia Commonwealth University for Individuals with Traumatic Brain Injury has been based on the individual placement approach. The authors view this as the best approach because it is the most normalized. The remainder of this chapter will address the development and implementation of the individual placement model of competitive employment.

Employment specialists: training and recruitment

A continuing challenge for the best supported employment programs has been the recruitment, training, and retention of quality staff. This has been a major problem for many programs because of limited funding, more complexity and diversity of workscope for employment specialists, and what at times is a highly frustrating quantity of work. The section which follows discusses the different work skills required.

It should be noted that most employment specialists work in programs for those with mental retardation and/or mental health problems. Only in recent years has supported employment begun to serve people with TBI. Current estimates indicate that fewer than 2,000 individuals with brain injury are receiving supported employment. Hence, very few training programs exist which specifically train employment specialists to assist individuals with TBI. What has been more popular is the multiday training sessions which university programs and hospitals offer to begin meeting this need. Unfortunately, this type of approach cannot come close to addressing the extraordinary occupational problems presented. Therefore, what has occurred is the pressing into service of existing employment specialists who know little about TBI, or utilizing TBI case-management staff who know very little about vocational service. These groups have begun to be cross-trained and, little by little, supported employment services are starting to emerge at different settings around the United States. Table 1 below suggests areas that should be covered when training supported employment professionals to serve individuals with TBI.

Training should also address information that is unique to serving people with TBI using a supported employment approach. This includes assessment and career development techniques, marketing and job development strategies, providing support and training on the job, long-term support services, and provision of case management services.

Table 1 Topics for Training Employment Specialists to Work For
         Individuals with Traumatic Brain Injury

Overview of TBI	Functions of the Brain
Definition of TBI	Frontal Lobe
Incidence	Temporal Lobe
Costs	Parietal Lobe
	Occipital Lobe
Types & Causes of Injury	**Medical Care**
Primary Damage	Acute Hospital Care
Secondary Damage	Post Acute Care
	Continuum of Care
Characteristics or Changes Resulting from TBI	**Health-Related Issues**
Physical	Depression
Sensory/Perceptual	Epilepsy
Communication	Sleep Disturbance
Cognitive	Substance Abuse
Behavioral	Medication and Side Effects
Impact on Family Systems	**General Counseling Techniques**
Family Members	Approaches
Income	When to Refer Out
Future	
Community Resources	**Leadership Skills**
National	Effective Communication
State	Conflict Resolution
Local	Problem Solving

The role of the employment specialist in helping persons with traumatic brain injuries return to work

Job coach. Trainer advocate. Employment specialist. These terms are often used interchangeably to describe the multifaceted work of a supported employment specialist. Employment specialists are paraprofessionals or professionals experienced in the fields of special education, rehabilitation counseling, psychology, and/or business and industry. In assisting persons with traumatic brain injuries to access jobs or return to work, the employment specialist takes on a variety of roles responding to the skills and support needs of the customer. The typical process involves the following steps: developing a customer profile, performing a career search that leads to employment, job-site training and support services, extended support services, and select case management. At the heart of this approach is empowering the customer to direct the process and participate in all activities to the fullest extent possible. The following section provides a brief description of the major components of supported employment and techniques for implementation.

Developing a customer profile

One of the first activities conducted after the person is referred for supported employment services is developing a customer profile. This involves gathering information from various sources about the customer's work preferences, strengths, and potential support needs.

Most individuals are referred and services are paid by state vocational rehabilitation counselors. The state vocational rehabilitation counselor plays an important role by providing information and insights about the customer's interests, abilities, personality propensities, learning potential, and career goals — often drawn from a basic vocational evaluation. If records are reviewed, they should be current. In addition, they should not be taken at face value since this may lead to preconceived notions about customer ability or the lack of it. The usefulness of records relative to the customer's vocational goal must also be taken into consideration.

Information from current records, like neuropsychological evaluations, supported employment questionnaires, and medical, psychological, educational, and past employment records are also utilized to help gain an insight into individual strengths and support needs.

At referral, if there is enough information and an agreeable direction for the job search has been established, then the next step is to move on to job development.

Select assessment approaches

Some customers and rehabilitation counselors, however, may feel that additional career planning is needed. Therefore, the supported employment provider should be able to recommend activities that will help further define the customer's vocational expectations. The employment specialist should review the possible activities with their customer and recommend a tailored approach that will render the most beneficial information for the career search. If possible, a visual reference combined with a clear and concise verbal explanation should be provided to promote customer understanding of these activities. A description of some possible assessment methods follow.

Situational assessment.   Situational assessments can give the customer an opportunity to work in actual employment settings. The customer explores interests, different types of work environments, preferences for instructional/training strategies, and potential job-site support needs. The customer selects from a variety of community-based assessment sites, the type of position he or she would like to experience, for what length of time, and the schedule of work hours. The customer also identifies cognitive, physical, and worker traits that he/she would like the employment specialist to assess during the situational assessment. Please refer to the section on Developing a Situational Assessment Site for more details.

Person-centered planning.   An alternative to assessing needs through testing and labeling is conducting "person-centered planning." This process focuses on abilities rather than deficits. It is planning the best quality future for a person based on strengths, preferences, and dreams for a life-style. During this process, a team works with the person to decide on a schedule of events and supports that will organize available resources to move toward the future.

Community assessment.   One useful technique in determining prefer-ences and functional ability is a community assessment conducted within the individual's neighborhood. Going out into the community provides indi-viduals with the chance to show the employment specialist what their skills are and what they like.

Informational interviews.   The customer may choose to provide names of people to contact who might have useful information. The interviews may be informal or structured. Interviewees might include previous employers, physicians, rehabilitation professionals, significant others, etc. The customer should be given the option to participate in the interview and encouraged to lead the session.

Vocational skills and knowledge assessment.   Some customers may desire to have their existing skills and knowledge as they related to a past or current specialized employment opportunity assessed (i.e., hair stylist, nurse, shoe repairman, etc.). In such cases, an assessment site is developed, and a con-sultant (person with the experience required) is hired to report on current skill level functioning. The Supported Employment staff would coordinate the effort and assess possible needs for accommodation. During this process, the focus is on examining acquired skills that are used proficiently. Note that these are not necessarily the things the person likes or is interested in doing. That's a separate issue.

Career search exercises.   Numerous tools, such as standardized career interest inventories and computerized vocational assessment instruments, are currently available to programs. Many of these tools are not specifically developed for persons with physical and cognitive disabilities, which must be taken into account when interpreting results. Nonetheless, the experience of actually working through a career search exercise with a customer can yield valuable assessment information in addition to helping the customer identify potential vocational interests.

Tours and interviews with local businesses.   This approach provides a valuable means for learning more about the customer's interests and abili-ties, as well as a particular occupation, industry, or employer. Observing the customer conducting an informational interview can yield valuable data on their interpersonal skills and communication abilities.

Complete profile

It is important to note that assessment should never be a lengthy process. Whenever the profile is complete, the career search should begin. Below is an outline for the contents of a customer profile. If more information is gleaned during the career search process, revise it.

- Customer identifies assets (skills and interests)
- Customer describes personal experiences (in terms of work, education, and other activities)
- Customer identifies work values or rewards expected
- Customer identifies work setting she/he will consider
- Customer, employment specialist, and vocational rehabilitation counselor determine how the above relate to career choice
- Customer secures references

The goal of assessment is to get a fair appraisal of where the customer initially wants to go and what she/he can offer to a business with or without reasonable accommodation. The person with a brain injury will obviously need more assistance than those with other disabilities in organizing this information for structural decision-making. This information should be reviewed and updated if needed.

Performing a career search

Once the employment specialist and customer have some ideas of the types of work tasks and/or employment settings that may best suit and satisfy the job seeker, a career search is started. Conducting the career search is not an easy process. It requires planning, a lot of legwork, and perseverance. During this stage the employment specialist and customer establish a plan to market the job seeker's talents to community businesses.

Some individuals may be able to perform existing job functions with little or no accommodation. Other people will not be able to perform the essential functions of existing jobs and will require that a job be carved for him or her. Regardless of the approach, the employment specialist will be responsible for utilizing a variety of approaches to discover the businesses that are willing to consider the individual for employment.

When meeting with potential employers, the employment specialist is initially concerned with finding out more about the businesses' needs and establishing rapport. During this process the employment specialist describes how he or she can refer potential candidates for consideration of employment if given additional insight into the business practices.

Additionally, he or she must be able to have a good sense of what types of work tasks the customer would not only be agreeable to performing, but also would be able to eventually perform independently after being provided with the necessary accommodations, including individualized job skills training. An understanding of how the person would be able to meld into the organization's social culture is another important consideration. The process of analyzing how a work opportunity and environment fit the customer can greatly influence the person's ability to retain employment.

Afterward, the compatibility analysis can be used to counsel the job seeker on how a particular opportunity may or may not be the right match for him or her. If the individual determines that he or she is indeed interested, then the next step is to arrange for an employment interview.

Job-site training and support services

Once employed, the new employee, employment specialist, and others, if chosen, will begin to brainstorm different support options and discuss the effectiveness and potential need for each. These options may be on or off site and might pertain to learning how to do the job effectively and safely, communicating with job-site personnel, handling issues outside of work, such as accessing transportation systems, depositing pay checks, etc. The new employee must be involved in choosing job-site supports. The employment specialist may actually provide the support or teach the employee how to access it. Some examples of supports are discussed below.

Educate job-site personnel

The customer may decide to discuss his/her condition with co-workers. This may release considerable tension for some people. Other customers may prefer not to disclose their disability, but may be in favor of a general educational inservice on disabilities to increase awareness and sensitivity among others. The Employment Specialist is available to discuss this option with management, and if they are agreeable, help make arrangements for a speaker.

Select instructional techniques

Most adults prefer to be self-directed learners. They refuse to be told what to do and have established preferences for learning. Additionally, when faced with a new learning situation, some customers may become anxious or uncomfortable. Therefore, the employment specialist must be prepared to take on various roles at the job-site, such as skills trainer and role model. Also, dependant upon the type of job, while the customer is learning how to do it, the employment specialist may actually perform some of the customer's job duties. This insurance for completing the expected workload keeps the boss satisfied and gives the new employee additional time to learn the job. Some instructional strategies are described below.

Modeling. This involves providing the learner with a correct and positive model to follow. The employment specialist demonstrates a series of steps in a task. This may be particularly useful when the employment specialist is attempting to train a client for jobs that require physical skills or develop behaviors which are difficult to describe or explain with words. Some skills and behaviors that may lend themselves best to modeling include loading and maintaining a film-processing machine, handling a customer complaint, asking for time off from work, and meeting coworkers.

Role-playing. This can be an effective training technique when the learner is attempting to develop a skill that involves face to face interactions. The role play can be used to explain how a situation should be handled and gives the learner a chance to practice a correct response. The learner and the employment specialist shift roles or choose to play the parts of others to encourage a fuller understanding of why a certain type of response is required. Each can take a turn at being the responder and observer of the situation at hand — role play with video feedback is ideal for clients with TBI.

Least prompts. This strategy is also referred to as a response prompt hierarchy, since the trainer progresses from the least amount of assistance (usually an indirect verbal prompt) to the most intrusive (usually a physical prompt) until one prompt stimulates a correct response.

Consideration should be given to selecting the most effective and preferred prompt by talking to the customer and trying out different sequences.

Regardless of the types of prompts selected, a latency period or time that the employment specialist will wait for the learner to respond before providing the next level of assistance should be established; for instance, 3 to 5 seconds time lapse is provided between prompts. People who have physical disabilities and/or a slowed rate of information processing, however, may require longer latency periods.

Time delay. In this procedure, the employment specialist chooses a single prompt that consistently allows the customer to perform the job duty correctly. At first, the prompt is given simultaneously with the request to perform the job task. Gradually, increasing amounts of time elapse before delivering the pre-selected prompt. This process is described in more detail in another section.

Create accommodations

The implementation of accommodations, such as compensatory strategies, adaptations and modifications, or restructuring of the work environment may enhance learning and promote his/her ability to perform independently at the job-site. Adjustments can be cognitively oriented, providing effective ways to remember what to do and how to do it; for example,

- A worksheet outlining the steps needed to balance a cash drawer
- A map that outlines a route to follow when cleaning apartment grounds

- Written detailed instructions to follow when cleaning plants

Other implementations may be used to compensate for lack of physical ability; for example,

- Providing a lap board for individuals involved in data entry to reduce ataxia
- Use of a stand to reduce unsteadiness in upright positions while sorting mail

Development and implementation of strategies may not occur unless the customer has difficulty learning a new task, shows variability in task performance, or is unable to meet the required production standard. Obviously, customer input will be very important in the selection of accommodations. Compensatory strategies and other accommodations are discussed in further detail in Chapter three.

Teach interpersonal skills

Some customers require a lot of support related to establishing and conducting interpersonal relations on the job. The employment specialist is available to help the customer in this area, if required. Modeling and role playing are two techniques that have been successfully used to assist customers in this area.

Sometimes, going to work and learning a new task can be very challenging. The inability to see immediate success can lead to frustration for the new employee. Frustration appears in many ways, such as verbal outbursts, throwing things, or even threats to quit a job. If this arises, the employment specialist is there to assist the new employee by providing encouragement, reinforcement, and scheduling of the learning at a pace compatible with the person's abilities. The employment specialist may teach techniques to help keep the outward signs of frustration at a minimum and manage these feelings. Understandably, an employer will only tolerate behaviors which appear rude or unusual for a limited amount of time. Therefore, it is important to immediately identify such difficulties and begin to provide immediate intervention.

Obtain performance feedback

The employment specialist should provide unbiased feedback to the customer on how she/he is progressing toward reaching the employer's performance standards. Generally, data are collected to substantiate progress. This data can also be used to determine the effectiveness of the training being provided.

To obtain and document the employer's perspective, the customer and employment specialist should use whatever protocol is in place for all employees, or in some instances, a tool, like a survey may be developed. If so, the questions should always be specifically related to job performance, and the format should be user-friendly (easy to understand and complete).

Design fading schedule

Eventually, the customer will begin to perform the job satisfactorily and the employment specialist will begin to reduce his or her presence at the job-site. This is a gradual process and is known as fading. The customer should give input into the design of the fading schedule by revealing what tasks he or she feels are mastered. This input should be taken into consideration when selecting the times of day to fade. Eventually, the employment specialist is absent from the job-site but keeps in touch at least a couple of times a month to review the employee's performance.

Customized job-retention services

It is important for the customer to learn to perform the job well. It is also crucial to keep it. A multitude of factors can influence the reliability of ongoing supports, such as a change in management or the way a job function is performed, the customer's transportation, or residential situation.

Therefore, it is critical that a method to keep abreast of how things are going both at and away from work is established. In supported employment, follow-up services are available throughout the duration of employment. During this phase, the employment specialist is no longer at the work site on a daily basis, but continues to have customer and employer contact and provides additional support services, if needed.

Choose performance indicators

As a proactive measure, the employment specialist monitors work performance throughout the period of employment. This is done through data that are collected during periodic job-site visits and through written supervisor evaluations that assess job production, and appropriate or inappropriate work behaviors. Workers may also fill out a self-evaluation form that provides the employment specialist with insight into the individual's perception of current job performance. One way to ensure that employment is stable is to gather information on how the customer is performing at work. Areas to monitor might include

- current job performance
- the employer's perceptions of performance
- effectiveness of compensatory strategies
- relations with job-site personnel
- job satisfaction
- any factors outside of work that affect job performance

Case management

Over the decades, supported employment providers have learned that the goal of vocational rehabilitation extends far beyond simply getting a job. Individuals must have access to a mix of services that are career oriented and unique to their specific needs and circumstances. Support services offered often extend beyond teaching the person (vocational) competencies at work. Support extends to assisting the person with community participation.

In providing supported employment services to individuals with traumatic brain injuries, the employment specialist functions in a number of roles. Along with job-site support and training, another role is that of a case manager. As a case manager, the employment specialist continually monitors and assesses an individual's employment situation and corresponding needs. Knowing how to respond effectively in a given situation is critical to a successful employment outcome. Therein lies the key to the employment specialist's role in helping persons with traumatic brain injuries return to work.

Throughout the duration of the supported employment relationship, the employment specialist may direct the client to a variety of resources, such as housing, transportation, reassessment of Social Security benefits, substance abuse treatment, marital and/or individual counseling, support groups for persons with traumatic brain injuries, and social/recreational programs, as indicated.

Developing a situational assessment site

It may be useful to conduct situational assessments for some job seekers prior to locating employment opportunities, particularly when an individual has had limited exposure to real work environments or the demands of working for an extended period of time. In most cases, these targeted tryouts or situational assessments are conducted within the private sector or paid temporary work. In other cases, federal work experience or university, hospital, and other job-sites are utilized to assess potential vocational strengths and interests. When conducting situational assessments, the employment specialist/job coach should be sure that the site(s) reflects the jobs that are available in the community. The assessments should last for at least a few hours in each setting, should provide information on the customer's job preferences, and assess ability to work across various conditions. Based upon an individual's time since injury, propensity for mental and physical fatigue, etc., shorter situational assessments are often considered as the first step in the transition to paid employment. Table 2 overviews the steps in establishing a situational assessment.

Table 2 Setting Up Situational Assessment Sites for Persons with
Traumatic Brain Injury

What do I look for?	What information does this give me?
Does this individual seem to show any preference across job types?	Providing several different job types for assessment may be useful in determining preferred job duties or work environments. If a job preference is established, it is more likely that a successful job match can be made. Remember that an individual with a severe brain injury often will not be able to say what he/she wants to do. Look for nonverbal signs, such as refusal to do certain types of work but not others, speed of work, and asking for excessive breaks
Does the consumer work more efficiently at specific times of the day?	It may be helpful to know whether the individual works more effectively during one portion of the day or another. His/her attention may be more focused and quality of work performance optimal. This information may be particularly useful when finding part-time positions, because difficult periods of the day could be avoided.
How long can the person work without stopping for a break?	Information that is gathered about an individual's stamina allows for specific job development. The employment specialist can then be sensitive to the frequency of breaks, amount of lifting, work speed required, etc. Stamina information may also indicate the length of the individual's work day. Someone with a low endurance might start out part-time and increase hours as endurance increases.
Does the individual respond positively or negatively to factors in the environment – noise, movement, objects, people, amount of space, etc.?	Individuals with severe impairment often have cognitive limitations or medical characteristics that affect how they respond to an environment. Sometimes these limitations are not obvious in nonwork settings. For example, a person who has difficulty walking may not do well in a cluttered work environment. He/she may also have difficulty if the job requires that work be done while walking but have no problem if the job is stationary. Another person who is easily startled may find excessive movement and noise problematic. Individuals may be able to make adaptions over time, but major limitations should be minimized with the job match. As discussed in Part A of this section, some consumers are attracted to work environments more than the actual job tasks. A situational assessment in an environment that appeals to them may provide the employment specialist with valuable data for job placement and vocational momentum for the client.

Table 2 (continued)   Setting Up Situational Assessment Sites for Persons with
Traumatic Brain Injury

What do I look for?	What information does this give me?
What types of prompts (verbal instructions, visual cues, sequenced pictorial instructions, etc.) does the individual respond to and what is the frequency?	Determining the types and frequency of prompts that an individual may need allows the employment specialist to develop instructional strategies for initial training. Instruction may then begin as soon as job placement occurs. This is valuable since individuals with severe impairment need to have consistent training from the first day of work to avoid error patterns of performance. In addition, if the person requires a high frequency of prompts, it will be important to note if the environment can maintain some frequency of prompts once the employment specialist fades from the site.

Setting up situational assessment sites for persons with traumatic brain injury

1. Review labor laws to ensure compliance.
2. Locate a source to purchase an individual insurance policy if requested.
3. Target jobs that represent actual jobs in the local community which may be available for individuals in supported employment programs.
4. Identify federal agencies, facilities, or businesses with targeted job positions.
   - Large federal agencies, universities, hospitals, nursing homes, etc. often have several departments within one facility that can be used for situational assessment sites.
   - These businesses may be preferable because they allow the employment specialist to make all contacts with only one personnel department. In addition, scheduling problems may be reduced by allowing staff to transport consumers to one central location for assessment.
5. Contact personnel director by phone.
   - Briefly describe the program, explaining the reason for contact.
   - Identify potential job types that may be appropriate for assessment.
   - Schedule an appointment to visit.
6. Visit the personnel director.
   - Describe supported employment and the purpose of a situational assessment.
   - Meet with the department supervisor(s) if possible.

- Schedule an appointment to observe in the identified depart-
  ment(s) to develop task analysis and job-duty schedules.
7. Visit the identified department(s).
   - Determine the jobs best suited for situational assessments.
   - Observe co-workers performing the jobs.
   - Develop a job-duty schedule and write task analyses.
8. Schedule the situational assessments.
   - Identify available times with the department supervisor(s).
   - Request at least four consecutive hours for each assessment.
   - Contact appropriate personnel, i.e., parents, teachers, facility staff,
     customers, etc.
   - Identify support staff to perform the assessments.
   - Send a copy of the schedule to the personnel director, department
     supervisor(s), parents, teachers, facility staff, etc.
9. Complete the following after the situational assessments.
   - Client Assessment Summary Form.
   - Thank-you letter to the Personnel Director and Supervisor(s).
   - Provide feedback to the customer, parents/guardians, teachers,
     facility staff, etc.

The following points represent items that may be important to observe
when conducting a situational assessment for an individual with a traumatic
brain injury. Remember that adaptations can be made after an individual
gets a job. In addition, skills can be acquired through training and repetition
of tasks. It is beneficial, however, to limit the need for extensive adaptations.
A good job match between the job seeker and position can do this and will
directly influence the number of intervention hours required before the
employment specialist can fade from the job-site or the amount of rehabilitation engineering that may be required.

Compensatory strategies and other accommodations

Compensatory strategies are effective techniques for teaching individuals with
traumatic brain injuries to regain functional skills for living and working more
efficiently. Compensatory strategies consist of external and internal aids used
to accomplish specific tasks. External aids are objects such as watches, grocery
lists, computer aids, alarm clocks, or appointment books that assist people
with remembering and organizing their environment. Internal aids include
techniques such as mental rehearsal, visual images, or mnemonics to assist
with memory or the comprehension of more abstract concepts. Techniques
such as personalized checklists and schedules ensure routine and minimize
the effects of memory and attention deficits. Although different types of strategies are presented in isolation, it is oftentimes the unique interplay and
sometimes a combination of approaches that lead to success at work.

Existing cues

The employment specialist should always be on the lookout for existing internal or external cues in a work environment that can foster independence and eliminate the need for introducing a new compensatory strategy on the job. Consider the following examples.

A patient transporter in a large hospital is able to find his way to the different areas of the building by following a color-coded paint strip on the wall of the hallways. The blue strip takes him to radiology, yellow goes to the laboratory, while red provides direction to the emergency room.

Another employee at a plastics-recycling center is required to sort various types of plastics into separate bins. He knows what bin to sort the container into by a number or letter code printed on the bottom of each item. The "S"-stamped containers go into the S bin, the containers without a stamp go into the bin that is not labeled, etc.

A stocker who works in a warehouse uses a computer printout that indicates where items are located and how many to retrieve.

Whenever considering a "job match" and during job-site training, the employment specialist should always use naturally occurring compensatory strategies. These cues can help enhance learning and promote independence at work; however, sometimes new compensatory memory strategies will need to be introduced at work, like those described below.

Internal strategies

Internal strategies require the use of mental support systems and do not rely on external devices.

Associations.   For example, a person can be taught to use associations or draw analogies between something that is being learned and what the learner already knows. Consider the employee who is taught to remember the proper pattern to follow when mopping a floor by associating this activity with how he mows the lawn.

Mnemonics.   Word mnemonics, like an acronym, may be designed and taught. For instance, an office clerk recalls her sequence of job duties by remembering that the letters in the word "CODE" stand for the order of the tasks to be performed. C is for clock in, O is for open mail, D is for deliver mail, E is for enter mail.

Word similarities and rhymes.   Word similarities may also be taught, like a maintenance man correctly recalling "left for loose" to remember how to loosen bolts or unscrew light bulbs.

Sometimes assisting the person with inventing sayings or rhymes that can help cue or recall what to do or what not to do may be helpful. Consider a young man working in a professional office setting as a file clerk who is experiencing difficulty maintaining an appropriate distance from females. He repeatedly attempts to hug female co-workers. To reduce this tendency he came up with the saying, "an arm's length away will let me stay." Afterward, he practiced saying this while extending his arm to give him a cue of the appropriate distance to stay away from females. This reminded him not only of what he needed to do, but also of the serious repercussions that would transpire if he failed to do it.

Verbal rehearsal. The transfer of information from short-to-long-term memory may be facilitated for some by verbally rehearsing instructions. For instance, an inventory control specialist sets up her workstation by stating aloud and talking herself through the process of "turn on the monitor, turn on the computer, enter my password, hit enter," and so on. Eventually she is taught to internalize this process by repeating the instructions a little more quietly each day until eventually they are repeated silently to herself.

Number chunking. Number chunking is another simple technique that involves recalling digits by reorganizing them into fewer elements. For instance, a file clerk may recall a number on a medical chart by recalling the digits one, seven, two, five as seventeen, twenty-five.

External strategies

External compensatory memory strategies involve the use of a device to augment the worker's abilities.

Checklists and flowcharts. One popular strategy is the use of checklists or flowcharts. This works particularly well when the task requires that the worker perform a specific sequence of steps. If, however, a task involves more complex learning or decisions need to be made based on a variety of inputs, a tree diagram may be used. For instance, a cashier might refer to a tree diagram in order to remember what procedures to follow when processing differing types of customer payments, such as checks vs. credit card vs. money order.

Reference manuals. Reference manuals help facilitate learning and also serve as a reference guide for the employee when the employment specialist is no longer on the job site. Consider a worker at a plant store and greenhouse who is responsible for providing maintenance to plants which have been housed at local businesses. The plants need to be cleaned to certain specifications according to the variety. A resource manual is developed which cross-indexes the plants by both common and phylum name. Each entry has a picture of the plant and written step by step instructions on the proper procedures to follow.

Location markers.   Location markers are another type of external strategy that can help remind a worker of where he or she is in task completion. For example, a warehouse worker was required to align and order shelf stock. Whenever he was called away from his immediate work area to fill a customer order or when he returned from break, he could not remember where on the aisle he had to go to continue his maintenance duties. To cue him about where he was in the process, he was taught to tie his bandanna around a post and use this to remember where to reinitiate his work activity.

Written cues such as labeling shelves and drawers are also another type of location marker. Highlighting can be used to facilitate visual scanning. For instance, a collections agent may use a colored marker to highlight data that are to be entered into a computer database, or a bookkeeper may keep her place on a document by placing a ruler directly under the text.

Maps.   Graphic representation of a work setting like a map may be used to assist a person with getting from point A to B. It may also be color-coded to show where work is performed and on what day. For example, a groundsman used a color-coded map to not only show him where to go, but also what duty to perform in that area on a given day; for example, "mow yellow areas on Monday, weed green areas on Tuesday, trim hedges on red areas on Wednesday," etc.

Scripts.   Scripts of written dialogues may also be used to prompt telemarketers on what to say to customers and teach proper telephone answering techniques or customer service skills. For example, a cashier was spending too much time talking to customers. Not only did the customer at the register appear annoyed by the small talk, but others in line did not like being delayed. The cashier felt he was just being friendly and could not understand why this was not considered good customer service. A script of what to say was posted near the register, and he referred to this repeatedly until he learned what to say at the start of a transaction, "Hello, how are you!" and when giving change and a receipt to the customer, "Thank you for shopping with us today."

Electronic devices.   Electronic devices are examples of external strategies. Some of the most commonly used electronic daily reminders are alarm watches and tape recorders. A watch with multiple alarms may cue individuals who have problems initiating task change.

Strategy development

Prior to developing a compensatory strategy, the employment specialist should determine if there is a need for one. This can be established by observing what the person is able to do without any additional assistance.

Indicators that may reveal the need for a strategy are when a person is silent and does not initiate an activity, has a difficult time performing a task, repeatedly asks for assistance, or makes the same mistakes over and over.

Once there seems to be a need for a strategy, then consideration of what other factors may be influencing performance outcomes should also be investigated. Environmental stimuli, like noise, lighting, constant movement of others around the person, or the effects of medications on cognitive abilities and rate of information processing may be contributing to the problem.

To increase their effectiveness, compensatory strategies must be functional and unobtrusive in the work setting, and they should be developed in conjunction with the employee who will be using them. Because they know about compensatory strategies that have been used successfully in the home, family members may also be especially resourceful. As people with traumatic brain injuries enter or return to employment, their independence and productivity can be greatly enhanced through the use of effective compensatory strategies.

Tips for developing compensatory strategies

- Σ The user must be involved in the design process
- Content must be individualized.
- Written strategies should use the minimal amount of text needed to prompt the response.
- Language must be directive and positive; for example, "Go to the breakroom," not "Do not forget to go to the breakroom."
- Strategies should blend into the work environment.
- Establish a location to keep a copy of the strategy at work where the employee will naturally come in contact with it.
- Keep additional copies of the strategies at the job-site, if strategies are taken home.
- Be aware that non-compliance may mean:
  - I forgot I had a strategy.
  - I feel stupid using this strategy.
  - I lost my strategy.
  - I was not involved in developing the strategy and do not think I need it.

Accommodations

In addition to using compensatory strategies there are a number of other ways businesses and/or employment specialists can help facilitate a successful work outcome for employees with a traumatic brain injury. These include making the environment accessible, restructuring jobs, modifying work schedules, rearranging work areas, and physical adaptations.

Accessible work areas. After a traumatic brain injury a person may encounter a change in their ability to walk and/or maintain their balance or experience weakness or paralysis on one or both sides of the body. An accessible workplace may be essential. Employment specialists can provide interested employers with information on how to make their site more accessible by providing information on the ADA, accessibility surveys, and information on tax credits for removal of architectural barriers. Some examples of how a business can make the workplace more accessible include installing automatic door openers or lever door knobs, leaving floors bare or using low-pile carpet and making sure that hallways are free of obstructions.

Job restructuring

This may be an appropriate accommodation for almost any functional limitation. Basically, this entails redistributing job functions, for instance, secondary tasks are reassigned to another worker; generally in exchange for another task. Employers may also approach this by considering what types of marginal functions a group of employees could stop doing and thereby have more time to spend in areas of expertise, while creating a work opportunity for another person.

Modified work schedules

Working forty hours a week of a routine or non-routine schedule can make employment difficult for some people. Splitting a full-time position into part-time work or adjusting a schedule to ease commuting problems can be very helpful for some individuals. Flexible schedules can allow someone with specific alertness cycles with a chance to work during his most energetic times of the day.

Allowing employees to take longer or more frequent breaks can also be helpful. This should not be additional break time but instead a longer break, for instance, fifteen minutes, or it could also be broken into three five-minute breaks. This may help counteract a decrease in energy or attention patterns, too.

Rearrangement of work areas

An employee's position in relation to equipment can have a profound impact on task performance. It is important to assist the person with finding the ideal position in front of the activity he or she is performing. For example, placing work materials on the left may be best if a person has problems with his right visual field. Modifying or redesigning a workstation to allow for easy access to work materials can often be done with ease.

Physical adaptations. Using physical adaptations, like trays or jigs, to keep material in place and improve work speed may be useful. For example, materials, such as electric staplers, rubber band holders, rubber finger tips, laminated work materials, and dycem matting increase work efficiency. Computer stations can be customized by adjusting the chair, work surface, monitor, and accessories.

Using systematic training strategies on a job site: a case study

The use of systematic behavioral training strategies on a job-site is critical to ensure that individuals with moderate to severe brain injuries learn the job duties correctly within a reasonable period of time.[2] A good behavioral training program should include reinforcement methods, specific prompting techniques, task analysis, data collection procedures, error correction, and criteria for fading the employment specialist's presence from the job-site.

There are several training strategies from which to select. Some of the prompting techniques include the system of least prompts, graduated guidance, and time delay. Consider the case of Mary, who was severely head injured in a automobile accident. She has serious memory deficits, is in a wheelchair, and has problems with organization and sequencing. This case study example is based on Mary's job as a laundry attendant. Her job duties of folding towels, pressing napkins, and pressing and folding pillowcases were taught using a time-delay procedure, a model prompt and reinforcement that consisted of social praise and coffee.

There are several critical components to a time-delay procedure. The trainer must select a prompt that will consistently assist the worker to perform the task correctly. Initially, the prompt is given simultaneously with the request to perform the task. Gradually, increasing amounts of time (usually seconds) are allowed between making the request to perform the task and providing the assistance/prompt to complete the skill correctly. Table 3 describes the intervention with Mary.

By pairing the prompt with the request to perform a skill, the worker is not allowed to make errors initially. The delay procedure allows the trainer to gradually fade assistance until the individual performs without prompting.

Using positive strategies to manage challenging behavior

John directs verbally abusive comments to his employment specialist and to his restaurant co-workers. Theresa whines continuously for no apparent reason while learning to perform her job as a laundry attendant at a large hospital. Sam engages in socially inappropriate actions by making sexual advances towards his employer at a merchandise warehouse.

Do these situations sound familiar with the clients with whom you work? Verbally abusive comments, crying on the job, and inappropriate social interactions are just a small sample of the behavior challenges that

Table 3 Time-Delay Procedures

Components of time delay	Mary's program components
1. Select prompt that the client responds to consistently.	1. Mary responded consistently to model prompts so this was selected.
2. Identify a reinforcer.	2. Mary responded well to verbal praise, but also received soda and candy at break as a reward for working.
3. Determine a preset number of delay seconds and trials.	3. One week of 0-second delay for all trials. Delay levels were increased when Mary met certain program objectives to 1, 3, 5, 6, 7, 8 seconds.
4. Determine a schedule of reinforcement.	4. Social praise on the average of every 3 responses, with break at the end of the task. Specific fading of reinforcement to the end of the task was planned as Mary met the program objective.
5. Specify an error correction procedure.	5. If 3 errors occurred in a row, the trainer went back to 0 seconds of delay for 10 trials. All errors were interrupted with a physical prompt.

may prevent persons with severe brain injury from obtaining and maintaining integrated employment. Low production rates, infrequent on-task behavior, and poor quality performance are additional challenging behaviors that represent major obstacles to maintenance of employment.

Individuals who work for natural reinforcers available on the work site, such as paychecks, supervisor/co-worker praise, positive written evaluations, pay raises, bonuses, and social interactions are more likely to be successful in supported employment and to not present challenging behaviors. However, many individuals with severe impairments have had little or no opportunity to experience these natural reinforcers within integrated employment settings and have difficulty managing their own behaviors. This presents a challenge to the employment specialist who must assist the worker in learning to function within the work environment.

It is the employment specialist's responsibility to teach the worker to respond to naturally occurring reinforcers and ultimately to engage in socially appropriate behaviors. Initially, it may be necessary to identify items that are not naturally occurring reinforcers for use on the job-site. In some instances, simply asking the new worker about likes and dislikes is sufficient. However, this method is frequently ineffective with employees experiencing brain injury residuals. The employment specialist should then observe the individual in a variety of settings and interview family members and other professionals (e.g., recreational specialists) familiar with the person's reinforcement needs. Regardless of the reinforcer identified, the employment specialist must consider several factors, including the timing, scheduling and eventual fading of the reinforcer to those that occur naturally on the job-site.

The key to success for supporting persons with behavior challenges in community-integrated employment settings has been a commitment by professionals to implement and be consistent with these techniques. Programs that have made this commitment find that they are able to serve individuals who have typically been excluded from the opportunity to obtain and maintain employment in community business settings. What follows is a discussion of program design.

Establishing a paycheck as a reinforcer

Many individuals with brain injury have had little exposure to money or have incomplete awareness that a paycheck represents money for work completed. This will present a problem to the employment specialist, since the paycheck is a naturally occurring reinforcer that obviously has the potential for providing a strong motivation for work. There are many different ways to teach a person the meaning of a paycheck. Some individuals may benefit from simply going with the employment specialist to cash the check and immediately use some of the money to buy a desired item. Another person may grasp the concept of a paycheck by marking off days on a calendar with the employment specialist indicating that payday will be approaching and that money will be used to buy an item. Still other individuals may learn the concept of a paycheck if a graph is made showing how many dollars are earned each day.

These ideas, however, may not work for the individual who does not realize that work results in money and that money can be used to buy things that he or she likes. Table 4 outlines a program designed for a young man who did not understand the relationship between working and earning a paycheck. John was refusing to work for large portions of the day when his employment specialist realized that she needed to implement a program to teach him the meaning of a paycheck.

Selecting a reinforcer

It is difficult to determine reinforcers for individuals with severe brain injuries in job-site settings. Unless an effective reinforcer can be determined, many workers will continue to be unsuccessful and fail to fully learn the job duties assigned to them. One way to systematically select a reinforcer is to use a multi-element design. In this program example, Mary had learned to fold towels as one of her job duties. However, she was not folding them to the production standard of the company.

The employment specialist wanted to select a reinforcer to use during a structured program to assist Mary in meeting her job requirements. She had three ideas that she thought might be effective, but was unsure of the best choice. The first idea consisted of using a timer to assist Mary in

Table 4 Relationship Between Working and Earning a Paycheck

Phase 1
- John's workday was divided into 5-minute intervals.
- He could earn a check on a card for working during the entire 5-minute interval.
- After he earned two checks on his card, John was given a nickel.
- John was able to spend the money that he earned during four designated break periods. There were pinball machines, video games, and a snack bar in his work environment.
- After two consecutive days of not refusing to work, Phase 2 of the program was implemented.

Phase 2
- John's workday was divided into 10-minute intervals.
- The other components of the program remained the same.
- After two consecutive days of not refusing to work, Phase 3 of the program was implemented.

Phase 3
- The workday continued to be divided into 10-minute intervals; however, John could only use his nickels to buy preferred items during two scheduled breaks. One occurred during the mid-point of the day and the other at the end of the day.
- After two consecutive days of not refusing to work, Phase 4 of the program was implemented.

Phase 4
- The workday was divided into 15-minute intervals.
- John no longer received a nickel as soon as he earned two checks on his card. Instead, the number of checks earned were totaled at the mid-point and end of the day prior to the two scheduled breaks. John was given the nickels he had earned at these times for spending.
- After two consecutive days of not refusing to work, the program moved to Phase 5.

Phase 5
- John's workday was divided into 20-minute intervals.
- During this phase, the checks John earned were totaled only at the end of the day for his nickels.
- After two consecutive days of not refusing to work, the program moved to Phase 6, etc.

Note: The length of the intervals before John received a check on his card for working was gradually increased. Use of the nickels eventually became unnecessary, as John began to receive money from his paycheck to spend every day. This type of program obviously takes a great deal of effort and planning by the employment specialist; however, John was able to understand the relationship between working, earning money, and receiving a paycheck by the end of the program.

From: Moon, M.S., Inge, K.J., Wehman, P., Brooke, V., and Barcus, J.M. (1990). *Helping persons with severe mental retardation get and keep employment: Supported employment issues and strategies.* Baltimore: Paul H. Brookes.

understanding the concept of folding a certain number of towels within a set time period. If Mary was successful, she would receive social praise from the employment specialist. The next idea incorporated the use of a picture diagram. The required number of towels to be folded within a ten-minute period was drawn on a card. If Mary met the number to be folded, she received a check on the card. Finally, the employment specialist thought it might be necessary to give Mary an edible reinforcer to increase her production. Mary would be told that she could earn candy in a cup that she could have at break if she worked faster. The strategy below was implemented by the employment specialist for reinforcer selection.

Using a Multi-Element Design to Select a Reinforcer

Program components	Mary's program
1. Select three reinforcers for observation.	1. The employment specialist selected candy, a picture check card, and a timer with social praise.
2. Determine the production standards by observing coworkers or by performing the task.	2. A co-worker could fold 25 towels within a ten-minute time period.
3. Determine the worker's production rate without reinforcement.	3. Mary was folding an average of 10 towels within a 10-minute time period.
4. Randomly assign a reinforcer to test intervals.	4. Twelve 10-minute test intervals were used for random assignment of the three reinforcers.
5. Implement the reinforcer and graph your results. Use the graph to determine if one reinforcers is more effective than the others.	5. The employment specialist told Mary prior to each trial that she could earn a specific reinforcer if she worked faster. The results were graphed for the 12 trials and it was determined that the most effective reinforcer was the use of the timer with social praise.

The most frequently asked questions and answers about individual supported-employment programming

Should individuals with behavior management problems be included in supported employment programs? Wouldn't it be better to get the behaviors under control in a sheltered workshop setting before community placement?

Attempting to eliminate behaviors prior to placement in the community may be an unsuccessful, as well as an unnecessary, program goal. For instance, many individuals with severe disabilities do not generalize well from one environment to another. Therefore, the staff of a sheltered workshop could work very hard to eliminate a behavior that would return as soon as the individual was exposed to a new environment. In addition, some behaviors may occur in one setting and not in another. The simple removal of an individual from the sheltered workshop and placement into a community work environment may eliminate the behavior problem. In summary, training should take place whenever possible within the natural environment in which the person is to ultimately function.

What reinforcers should I use on a job-site for my behavior management programs?

The best reinforcers to utilize during job-site training are those that occur naturally in the work environment. This might include the paycheck, co-worker praise, or supervisor praise. The employment specialist must take time for observation of the work site to identify naturally occurring reinforcers as well as naturally occurring times for delivery. For instance, the supervisor may walk by the consumer's workstation on a regular schedule; this contact with the supervisor could be incorporated into a behavior management program.

However, sometimes it is necessary to consider using more tangible reinforcers, such as magazines, coffee, money, or food items. The employment specialist should try to use these items in a nonintrusive way to not draw attention to the client. In addition, tangible items should only be used on a job-site if a procedure has been developed to fade use to naturally occurring reinforcers.

When should reinforcement be delivered?

The timing of reinforcement is critical. All reinforcement should be given quickly and immediately following the occurrence of the appropriate worker behavior. Sometimes it may not be feasible to deliver a particular reinforcer immediately, particularly in the case of tangible reinforcers. In these situations, exchangeable reinforcers such as points, tokens, or checks are immediately provided and exchanged later, i.e., a soda during break time.

The employment specialist must also determine a schedule of reinforcement which dictates how often the item will be delivered. During initial instruction, a continuous schedule is generally recommended. This means that the worker receives reinforcement for each behavior or step of a task that is performed correctly. As the worker's performance increases or improves, the reinforcement is gradually decreased to a predetermined period of time or number of correct responses. As the worker performs the behavior or task, the reinforcement schedule should be gradually changed until the individual is reinforced on a natural schedule for the workplace. The timing and scheduling of reinforcement always should be based on the skill level of the worker and demands of the environment.

How can I collect data on behavior management programs when I am already busy with skill acquisition programs?

Data collection can be problematic for the busy employment specialist who is trying to track several programs at one time. The solution is to develop innovative ways to collect data that fit into the daily routine. Frequency counts should be collected using golf counters or markings on a piece of tape attached to the employment specialist's wrist. One job trainer used the change in his pockets to take a frequency count by transferring coins from one pocket to another when the targeted behavior occurred. This information can then be recorded on a formal data sheet during break time or at the end of the day.

How can I implement a behavior management program when I am already busy with all the other demands of the work environment?

The employment specialist can determine the most appropriate time of the day for program implementation by observing the events that occur on the job before and after a behavior occurs. For instance, the employment specialist may determine that the worker swears loudly whenever he has to perform a particular job duty. Therefore, the behavior strategy would be implemented during this time period.

However, if no particular time of day can be identified, several decisions must be made. For instance, the employment specialist must determine if it is possible to use the behavior strategy throughout the day whenever the identified problem occurs. This would be the strategy of choice since it is important to be consistent if behavior is to change. If the work environment is such that this is impossible, the employment specialist should identify blocks of time during the day in which intensive programming can be provided. As the individual learns his or her job and begins to perform to job-site expectations, the program can be used in other portions of the day.

How do I know if my program is working, and when should I make changes in my behavior management strategies?

Prior to program implementation at the job-site, a baseline period of performance should be established; this is used as a comparison measure with program implementation data. As long as a steady decrease in negative behaviors or an increase in appropriate behaviors and speed of performance is noted, the employment specialist should continue with programming. No changes over a series of days indicate that modifications are necessary and might include the use of another reinforcer or program strategy to include compensatory measures. The employment specialist is cautioned to remember that maladaptive behaviors will often return on a short-term basis in the middle of a behavior management program. This is especially true as program criteria are changed, such as increasing the length of time for appropriate behavior to occur before delivery of the reinforcer. In this instance, consistency and patience are important. The employment specialist may need to revert to a previous program level and increase program requirements at a slower rate.

Job retention/follow-along

Once the client with TBI has been successful and consistent at independently performing the job duties, meeting production standards, and is successful interacting with persons and using other appropriate behaviors in the work environment, the employment specialist gradually fades his/her presence from the job-site. Once stabilization has been determined, the individual moves into the follow-along phase of supported employment.

From a state rehabilitation or legislated viewpoint, the term stabilization refers to a point in time when time-limited funding is terminated and extended services funding begins. The guidelines for determining stabilization differ from state to state. For example, in Virginia, stabilization occurs "when average staff intervention time falls below 20 percent of the individual's work hours for 30 days of employment." For purposes of funding, it is important that a program be cognizant of how to determine stabilization. However, for the purpose of this text the term is not to be used in reference to the point at which funding mechanisms change, but to indicate when an individual has reached a job performance status that moves them into the follow-along phase of supported employment. An individual will be placed into follow-along status on the specific date when employment specialist intervention is no longer required on the job-site.

Follow-along is the job maintenance or retention phase of the supported employment model. Follow-along may be defined as an ongoing assessment and monitoring of the individual's work performance and behaviors/factors that require collecting information/data, making observations, and providing advocacy in an effort to anticipate problematic situations and to offer proactive intervention. Additional intervention and support services are available for the duration of the individual's employment. During this phase, the employment specialist is no longer at the work site on a daily basis, but continues to have scheduled contacts with the individual and employer.

Planning extended services

Follow-along activities are provided to enhance the likelihood of an individual maintaining employment and should incorporate a systematic approach that includes ongoing monitoring of the individual's work performance and assessing factors outside of employment, i.e., case management issues that may affect the individual's work performance (transportation usage, family dynamics, medication management, etc.). To ensure continuous employment, a plan must be devised that enables the employment specialist to gather current data/information that will provide continual assessment of the following areas to be monitored:

1. The individual's dependability;
2. The individual's current job performance;
3. The employer's current perception of the individual's job performance;
4. Appropriateness of current or need for new compensatory strategies, adaptations, or modifications;
5. Dynamics of interpersonal job-site relations;
6. Changes in the individual's daily routine, job duties, or work environment;
7. The individual's level of satisfaction with the employment; and
8. Factors outside of work which may adversely affect satisfactory job performance if left unattended.

This requires proactive planning and a useful tool for recording information, data, and observations during future follow-along contacts.

Follow-along plan of action meeting

During the planning phase, a follow-along plan of action provides a format that may be useful in reviewing information obtained during job-site training and future follow-along contacts to assist in forecasting the development of a proactive follow-along schedule and in identifying areas for monitoring during this follow-along component of supported employment. At the point of stabilization, the employment specialist and program manager meet to determine the follow-along plan of action. Once the plan of action is devised, the follow-along performance review is completed during the scheduled follow-along contacts.

During the initial plan of action meeting, information from daily performance baselines, reviews, and supervisor evaluations are examined. This requested information is recorded on the plan of action according to the following step-by-step instructions:

Follow-Along Plan of Action

I. Placement Information

A. Client: _____   D. Position: _____
B. Employer:_____   E. Date of Hire:_____
C. Schedule: _____   F. Wage: _____
G. Date of Employer's Performance Review: _____

II. Employment Updates

The employment update consists of the completion of the Job Update, Client Update, and Supervisor- and Self-Evaluation forms on a scheduled basis. Employment update forms are completed during the 3rd and 6th month of employment and then every 6 months throughout the term of employment. The Supervisor- and Self-Evaluation forms, however, as previously mentioned during job-site training are also completed at two weeks and 1 month post-placement.

The Job Update Form gathers current information on wages earned, hours employed, and level of integration. The Client Update form collects information on current vocational rehabilitation case status, residential situation, mode of transportation, and types and amounts of financial aid.

Supervisor- and Self-Evaluations are also completed as part of the employment update. On the Plan of Action Form, using the consumer's date of hire as day one, determine the date that the employment updates are due.

During future planning meetings, write in the date on the plan of action of when the employment update is completed. Examples of the employment update forms and how to complete each follow.

	Employment Update	
	Due	Completed
3rd month	_____	_____
6th month	_____	_____
12th month	_____	_____
18th month	_____	_____
24th month	_____	_____
30th month	_____	_____

III. Attendance/Punctuality

A. Record the number of days the client was absent during job-site training and a brief explanation of why the individual (he/she) was absent.

B. Record the number of days the client was untimely for arrival, breaks, and departure from work during job-site training.
C. Based on the above, determine whether or not this is an area of concern to be monitored closely during follow-along. Circle *Yes* or *No*.
Absent #
Arrival _____ Breaks _____ Departure _____
Area of concern? yes/no

IV. Job Performance Information

A. List the job duties the individual performs.
B. Record baseline quality and production % of standards.
C. Review training data and check off areas that need to be monitored during follow-along visits.
D. Record day and time this duty may be observed.
E. Asterisk duties performed which require the use of a compensatory strategy.

During future planning meetings, write in the Month/Year data were collected regarding job duty performed.

Month/Yr Observed	(A) Job Duties	(B) Skill Acq./Quality Production/ Prod. Qual.	(C) Area of Concern	(D) Schedule
_____1.				
_____2.				
_____3.				
_____4.				
_____5.				
_____6.				
_____7.				
_____8.				

*Asterisk duties which require use of compensatory strategy. Circle asterisk if there is a need to check consistency in use.

V. Compensatory Strategies

Compensatory Strategies   Consistency in Use

1.
2.
3.
4.
5.

VI. Behavioral Information

A. Using past incident reports, categorize similar incidents and record type.
B. Record the number of occurrences.
C. Indicate the date of the last incident.
D. Check off areas of concern that need to be monitored during follow-along visits.

(A) Incidents	(B) # Occurrence	(C) Date	(D) Area of Concern
1.			
2.			
3.			
4.			
5.			
(E) Other: _____			

VII. Work Environment

A. Have any of the items listed 1 – 6 changed since employment?
   Y = Yes,   N = No.   Circle one.
B. If "Yes," approximately how many times?
C. What was the date of the last change?
D. Is this an area of concern?

	(A) Yes/No	(B) Frequency	(C) Date	(D) Area of Concern
1.	Schedule	Y N		
2.	Supervisor	Y N		
3.	Co-Workers	Y N		
4.	Job Duties	Y N		
5.	Work Station	Y N		
6.	Other:			

VIII. Sources of Information

A. List names and position/title or relationship of those individuals to be contacted during follow-along visits.
B. Indicate what information the individual listed can provide.
C. Write any special notes regarding interaction with those individuals: co-workers, management, supervisors, family, etc.

(A) Name/Title	(B) Information	(C) Notes
1.		
2.		
3.		
4.		

IX. Case Management

A. List current case management issues.
B. Record plan of action. Also, list possible case management issues which should be monitored closely during follow-along.

(A) Issues	(B) Plan of Action
1.	
2.	
3.	
4.	
5.	

X. Notes:

Use this space to record any additional information vital to providing proactive follow-along services not previously taken into consideration or stated.

_____

_____

_____

_____

XI. Proposed Follow-Along Schedule

Based on the information reviewed, indicate the proposed date for a follow-along visit to take place using (/) symbol on calendar. Once the visit has taken place, put an (x) symbol on the calendar. Use an asterisk (*) to indicate dates that consumer updates are due. Circle the asterisk when the update is complete. Schedule the next update meeting. Indicate date with an (M) on the calendar. Update the plan of action on a scheduled basis using information collected during follow-along performance reviews and past plans of action.

MONTH:							MONTH:							MONTH:						
S	M	T	W	T	F	S	S	M	T	W	T	F	S	S	M	T	W	T	F	S

Level _____   Level _____   Level _____

During future plan of action meetings, information from previous follow-along plans of action and performance reviews is assessed to record the information requested. Based on the information and data reviewed, the employment specialist proposes the first month's follow-along schedule to meet the specific needs of the individual.

The following factors will assist in determining the initial appropriate level of follow-along:

- Time post-stabilization.
- Attendance and punctuality during job-site training.
- Consistency in job performance during job-site training and use of compensatory strategies.
- Number and type of incidents that occurred during training related to medication or self-medication.
- Current case management needs, stability of living situation, and relationships outside of work.
- Emotional stability of client particularly if the individual is a risk for depression, anxiety attacks, or substance abuse.
- The support system available in the work/home environment.
- The perceived need for contact as identified by the individual and employer.

During the first month post-stabilization, the employment specialist should schedule a visit to the job-site at a minimum of two contacts per week. Based on the outcome of the following visits, the employment specialist and program manager meet to establish what level of follow-along intensity to provide.

Level III: A minimum of two contacts per week with the client and employer.
Level II: A minimum of one contact per week.
Level I: The legal and clinical minimum of one contact every two weeks

The employment specialist should record the proposed schedule on a master monthly follow-along calendar. This will help prevent overlap of schedule times to visit various job-sites. If another employment specialist or the program manager has to cover follow-along contacts due to one specialist's absence, vacation, or other training demands, the master schedule will be easily available and continuity of services can be provided.

References

1. McMordie, W.R., Barker, S.L., and Paolo, T.M. (1990). Return to work (RTW) after head injury. *Int. Rehabil. Med.*, 2, 17–22.
2. Parenté, R. (1994). Effects of monetary incentives on performance after traumatic brain injury. *NeuroRehabilitation*, 4:3, 198–203.
3. Greenspan, A.I., Wrigley, J.M., Kresnow, M., Branche–Dorsey, C.M., and Fine, P.R. (1996). Factors influencing failure to return to work due to traumatic brain injury. *Brain Injury*, 10, 207–218.
4. Brooks, N., McKinlay, W., Symington, C., Beattie, A., and Campsie, L. (1987). Return to work within the first seven years of severe head injury. *Brain Injury*, 1, 113–127.
5. Wehman, P., West, M., Kregel, J., Sherron, P., and Kreutzer, J. (1995). Return to work for persons with severe traumatic brain injury. A data–based approach to program development. *J. Head Trauma Rehabil.*, 10:1, 27–39.
6. Thomsen, I.V. (1984). Late outcome of very severe blunt head trauma: a 10–15 year second follow–up. *J. Neurol. Neurosurg. Psychiatry*, 47, 260–268.
7. Lezak, M. (1986). *Neuropsychological Assessment*, 2nd ed. New York: Oxford University Press.
8. Sale, P., West, M., Sherron, P., and Wehman, P. (1991) An exploratory analysis of job separations from supported employment for persons with traumatic brain injury. *J. Head Trauma Rehabil.*, 6:3, 1–11.
9. West, M. (1996). Assisting individuals with brain injuries to return to work: new paradigms of support. *J. Voc. Rehabil.*, 7, 143–149.
10. Weddell, R., Oddy, M., and Jenkins, D. (1980). Social adjustment after rehabilitation: A two-year follow-up of patients with severe head injury. *Psychol. Med.*, 10, 257–263.
11. Rappaport, M., Herrero–Backe, C., Rappaport, M.L., and Winterfield, K.M. (1989). Head injury outcome up to ten years later. *Arch. Phys. Med. Rehabil.*, 70, 885–893.
12. Rao, N., Rosenthal, M., Cronin–Stubbs, D., Lambert, R., Barnes, P., and Swanson, B. (1990). Return to work after rehabilitation following traumatic brain injury. *Brain Injury*, 4, 49–56.
13. Wehman, P., Kreutzer, J., West, M., Sherron, P., et al. (December, 1989). Employment outcomes for persons following traumatic brain injury: Preinjury, postinjury and supported employment. *Brain Injury*, 4, 397–412.
14. Wehman, P., Kreustzer, J., West, M.D., Sherron, P., Zasler, N.D. Groah, C.H., Stonnington, H.H., Burns, C.T., and Sale, P.R. (1990). Return to work for persons with traumatic brain injury: A supported employment approach. *Arch. Phys. Med. Rehabil.*, 71, 1047–1052.

15. Wehman, P., Sherron, P., Kregel, J., Kreutzer, J., Tran, S., and Cifu, D. (1993). Return to work for persons following severe traumatic brain injury: Supported employment outcomes after five years. *Am. J. Phys. Med. Rehabil.*, 72, 355–363.

16. Albin, J. and Slovic, R. (1992). *Resources for Long-term Support in Supported Employment.* Eugene, OR: University of Oregon, The Employment Network.

17. West, M. and Parent, W.S. (1995). Community and workplace supports for individuals with severe mental illness in supported employment. *Psychosoc. Rehabil. J.*, 18:4, 13–24.

18. West, M., Revell, W.G., and Wehman, P. (1992). Achievements and challenges I: A five–year report on consumer and system outcomes from the supported employment initiative. *J. Assoc. Persons Sev. Hand.*, 17, 227–235.

19. West, M. (1995). Choice, self–determination, and VR services: Systemic barriers for consumers with severe disabilities. *J. Voc. Rehabil.*, 5, 281–290.

20. Moon, S., Goodall, P., Barcus, M., and Brooke, V. (Eds.), (1986). *The supported work model of competitive employment for citizens with severe handicaps: A guide for job trainers* (rev. ed.), Richmond: Virginia Commonwealth University, Rehabilitation Research and Training Center.

21. Kregel, J., Wehman, P., Revell, W.G., and Hill, M. (1990). Supported employment in Virginia: 1980–1988: In F.R. Rusch (Ed.), *Supported employment: Models, methods and issues* (pp. 15–29). Baltimore: Paul H. Brookes Publishing Co.

22. Bellamy, G.T., Rhoades, L.E., Boubeau, P.E., and Mank, D.M. (1986). Mental retardation services in sheltered workshops and day activity programs: Consumer benefits and policy alternatives. In F.R. Rusch (Ed.), *Competitive employment issues and strategies* (pp. 257–272). Baltimore: Paul Brookes Publishing Co.

23. Borbeau, P. (1985). Mobile work crews. In P. Wehman and J. Kregel (Eds.), *Supported employment for persons with disabilities.* New York: Human Sciences Press.

24. Mank, D., Rhodes, L., and Bellamy, G.T. (1986). Four supported employment alternatives. In W. Kiernan and J. Stark (Eds.), *Pathways to employment for adults with developmental disabilities.* Baltimore: Paul Brookes Publishing Co.

25. Rhoades, L.E. and Valenta, L. (1985). Industry based supported employment. *J. Assoc. Persons Sev. Hand.*, 10, 12–20.

26. O'Bryan, A. (1989). The small business supported employment options for persons with severe handicaps. In P. Wehman and J. Kregel (Eds.), *Supported employment for persons with disabilities.* New York: Human Science Press.

27. Boles, S., Bellamy, G., Horner, R., and Mank, D. (1984). Specialized training program: The structured employment model. In S.C. Paine, G.T. Bellamy, and B. Wilcox (Eds.), *Human-services that work.* Baltimore: Paul Brookes Pub. Co.

Index

A

ABLE, see Adult Basic Learning Exam
ABPP/ABCN, see American Board of
        Professional Psychology/ American
        Board of Clinical Neuropsychology
Abstract thinking, 22
Abusive language, 26
Academic achievement, 78
Academic environment, difficulty of persons
        with brain injury in, 144
Acceleration injury, 21
Accommodation program, 136
ACRM, see American Congress of Physical
        Medicine and Rehabilitation
ADA, see Americans with Disabilities Act
Adaptive reasoning, 36, 62
Adult Basic Learning Exam (ABLE), 168
Affirmative industry, 177, 181
Agency-based supports, 188
Agitation, 22
Agnosia, 72
Agraphia, 72
Alarm clocks, 219
Alcohol
    abuse, 71, 107
    avoidance of following TBI, 122
    effects of after injury, 68
Alexia, 72
American Board of Professional
        Psychology/American Board of
        Clinical Neuropsychology
        (ABPP/ABCN), 39, 41
American Congress of Physical Medicine and
        Rehabilitation (ACRM), 44
American Psychological Association (APA),
        41, 44, 76
Americans with Disabilities Act (ADA), 130,
        183, 184

Amnesia, 64, 97
Anger, 12, 24
    management, 104
    outbursts, 22
    transition, 26
Anticipatory awareness, 109
Anxiety, 12, 99
APA, see American Psychological
        Association
Aphasia, 72, 103
Appetite
    change, 60
    poor, 99
Applied behavior analysis, 28
Apraxia, 72
Assistive technology, use of in vocational
        rehabilitation of persons with
        traumatic brain injury, 129–160
    adapting work environments, 152–158
        analyzing and modifying tasks to
            improve performance, 153
        ergonomic considerations to improve
            speed and endurance, and avoid
            fatigue, 153–158
        understanding workflow and
            influence of associated operations,
            153
    augmenting academic and vocational
        activities, 143–152
        electronic aids, 146–152
        executive administrative function, 144
        verbal and written expressive function,
            144–146
        verbal and written recapture function,
            144
    behavioral concerns in workplace,
        136–138
        issues of integration, 136–137
        risk management, 137–138

job restructuring, 224
modified work schedules, 224
rearrangement of work areas, 224–225
strategy development, 222–223
tips for developing compensatory
    strategies, 223
customized job-retention services,
    215–219
case management, 216
choosing performance indictors, 215
developing situational assessment site,
    216–218
setting up situational assessment sites
    for persons with traumatic brain
    injury, 218–219
description of supported employment
    models, 204–207
enclaves in industry, 206
entrepreneurial model, 206–207
individual placement model, 205
mobile work crews, 205–206
employment specialists, 207–212
complete profile, 211
developing customer profile, 209
performing career search, 211–212
role of employment specialists in
    helping persons with traumatic brain
    injuries return to work, 208
selecting assessment approaches,
    209–210
frequently asked questions and answers
    about individual supported-
    employment programming, 230–233
collecting data on behavior
    management programs, 231
delivery of reinforcement, 230–231
implementing behavior management
    program, 231
job retention/follow-along, 232–233
reinforcers used on job site, 230
success of program, 232
initiating and maintaining supported
    employment program, 202–204
natural supports, 203
self-determination and choice, 204
job-site training and support services,
    212–215
creation of accommodations, 213–214
design of fading schedule, 215
education of job-site personnel, 212
obtaining performance feedback,
    214–215
selection of instructional techniques,
    212–213
teaching of interpersonal skills, 214

planning extended services, 233–239
using positive strategies to manage
    challenging behavior, 225–229
using systematic training strategies on job
    site, 225
Supported Employment Program at Virginia
    Commonwealth University for
    Individuals with Traumatic Brain
    Injury, 207
Switchboard operator, 32
Symbol Digit Modalities Test, 52

T

Task
    analysis, 225
    lists, sequenced, 195
Tax-exempt status, 179, 182
TBI, see Traumatic brain injury
Technology Related Assistance for
    Individuals with Disabilities Act, 129
Temporal lobes, 17
Test
    construction, 40
    hypothesis, 42
    results, translating, 40
    scores, interpreting, 43
Thematic Apperception Test, 12
Therapeutic contracting, 106
Time-delay procedure, 225
Tourette's Syndrome, 71
Trades, visual skills necessary in, 34
Trail Making Test, 38
Training
    consultant, community, 188
    job skills, 205
    on-the-job, 37, 178
    program, implementing co-worker, 191
    punctuality during job-site, 238
    requirements, 197
    self-awareness, 114
    vocational, 173
    work adjustment, 178
Transferable skills assessment, 165, 166
Transportation
    assistance, 178
    usage, 233
Traumatic brain injury (TBI), 1, 163, 177
    choosing placement model in, 186
    concentration deficits after, 32
    employment program for survivors of, 162
    group work with clients with, 121
    life function affected by, 31
    mechanisms of, 20

discharge planning, 9–10
treatment planning and monitoring of
progress, 8–9
vocational re-entry planning, 11
questions to ask neuropsychologist, 45–49
needs of neuropsychologist, 45–46
what is helpful to vocational
rehabilitation professional, 46–49
traditional psychological vs.
neuropsychological evaluations,
11–15
comprehensive neuropsychological
evaluation, 13
cost, 13–14
neuropsychological evaluation, 12–13
psychological evaluation, 11–12
requesting rehabilitation-oriented
report, 14–15
utilizing neuropsychologist in vocational
planning, 39–45
poorly qualified specialists, 42–44
practitioners of neuropsychological
services, 39–40
selection recommendations, 44–45
theoretical orientations in
neuropsychology, 42
training background of
neuropsychologist, 41–42
Vocational rehabilitation (VR), 202
Vocational skills, 210
Vocational training, 173

Volunteer work, 105
VR, see Vocational rehabilitation

W

Walk before you run argument, 181
Wechsler Adult Intelligence Scale, 12, 30, 52,
61, 168
Wechsler Memory Scale, 38
White matter, 16
Wisconsin Card Sorting Test, 52, 61
Woodcock Johnson Psychoeducational
Achievement Battery, 168
Word
-finding difficulties, 54
prediction software, 146
-processing software, 146
similarities, 220
Work
activity, accuracy of, 153
adjustment training, 178
environments, 152, 236
-related impairments, 153
sample performance, 175
schedules, modifying, 223, 224
trials, 114
values, 164, 174
Worker behaviors, 175
Working memory, 18
Written language, 55